Essential Yoga With Props

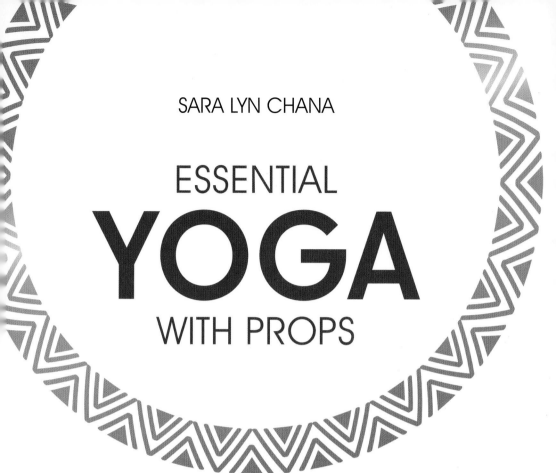

SARA LYN CHANA

ESSENTIAL
YOGA
WITH PROPS

Enhance Every Pose for
Full-Body Mobility and Flexibility

Meyer & Meyer Sport

British Library of Cataloguing in Publication Data
A catalogue record for this book is available from the British Library

Originally published as: *Yoga mit Hilfsmitteln*, © 2023 by Meyer & Meyer Verlag, Aachen, Germany

Essential Yoga With Props
Maidenhead: Meyer & Meyer Sport (UK) Ltd., 2025
ISBN 978-1-78255-276-5

Aachen, Auckland, Beirut, Cairo, Cape Town, Dubai, Hägendorf, Hong Kong, Indianapolis, Maidenhead, Manila, New Delhi, Singapore, Sydney, Tehran, Vienna

Member of the World Sport Publishers' Association (WSPA), www.w-s-p-a.org
Printed by Print Consult GmbH, Munich, Germany
Printed in Slovakia

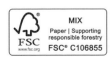

ISBN: 978-1-78255-276-5
Email: info@m-m-sports.com
www.thesportspublisher.com

▶Contents

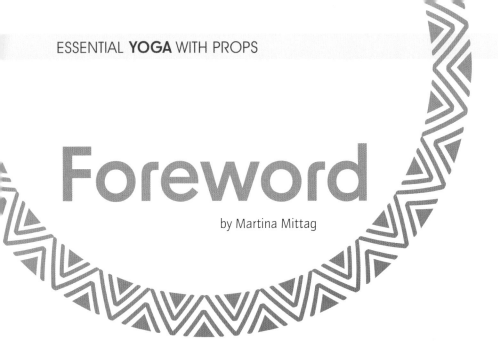

Foreword

by Martina Mittag

If you're holding this book in your hands, you might be a yoga teacher seeking ideas and instructions on using yoga props. Alternatively, you may be a yoga practitioner wondering about the possibilities for the props you might have purchased as part of a set with a mat, now collecting dust because, apart from two or three standard exercises, you're unsure how to use them.

When I think back to my childhood, I still vividly remember some rather amusing yoga books on the shelf at home. It was a time when women wore fine stockings under leotards, and wiry men, usually middle-aged, were depicted in short gymnastics shorts. Props were neither used nor mentioned. At best, there might have been a yoga mat or a blanket as a prop.

On my first visit to South India in 2001, I spent time in a yoga ashram, where regular hikes to one of the surrounding mountains were organized. The journey began at 3:30 am in the middle of the night, ascending the mountain through the twilight. I was pretty impressed by the pace set by our Swami. After about two hours without a break, we all reached our destination, quite sweaty. But instead of comfortably sitting down to contemplate the sunrise, our Swami announced, "And now, Surya Namaskar!"

Seriously, our Swami instructed us to practice the Sun Salutation right then and there! We all exchanged amused and slightly bewildered glances. Surely, this had to be a joke? When we mentioned that we didn't have any yoga mats, the Swami dismissed our concerns promptly and assertively, stating in a tone that brooked no objection: "For a Yogi, a stone is like a bed! Surya Namaskar! Immediately!" And so, somewhat bewildered and hesitant, we embarked on our twenty-one Sun Salutations. In retrospect, it was a very intense experience. Surprisingly, the absence of yoga mats didn't matter after the first two rounds. Yoga without anything—it works!

Why use props?

Before the influential Indian yoga teacher B.K.S. Iyengar introduced a range of props to the yoga community, they weren't widely used. In his widely recognized book, Light on Yoga,[1] released in 1966, he showcased yoga poses without the props now commonly associated with Iyengar Yoga. It wasn't until the mid-to-late 1980s that props gradually became recognized.

It was during that time that the general use of props began, though not in the variety we know today. It started with mats specifically designed for yoga, and even in this category, there is a vast selection available today. Very lightweight, thin mats for traveling, non-slip mats for beach poses and flows, thick mats for yoga practices primarily done on the floor (regenerative practice), and sheepskin mats, which are meant for relaxation—all distinguished by organic and ecological labels. In addition, there is plenty of poorly made "brand junk"—mats that are too slippery or smell unpleasantly of chemicals, hardly suitable for yoga practice.

The situation is similar with yoga or meditation cushions. There is remarkable diversity here regarding material, size, and shape. What appeared on the market over time were yoga blocks, straps, and, eventually, yoga bolsters. And let's not overlook the trusty "old" woolen blankets with their own set of requirements. They shouldn't be too slippery, they need to fold easily, and they must be of a particular volume when used for supporting the hips, shoulder girdle, or knees. Cozy fleece blankets, though perfect for covering up during deep relaxation, don't quite cut it as props for active practice.

A downright "battle of materials" has emerged over the last three decades.

What makes Hatha Yoga so unique is that there are always areas that can be controversial—free from the necessity of having to conform to a specific perspective.

"It depends" is what international yoga colleagues usually say in yoga seminars when asked a "Yes/No," "Right/Wrong," or "For/Against" question. It depends on the perspective from which we consider the respective topic.

My yoga training includes a seminar on the topic "Yoga Props—Assistance in Yoga Practice." At the start, participants are tasked with creating a pros and cons list in groups. Their goal is to identify arguments in favor of using props like blocks or straps and delve into the critical aspects associated with them.

There are plenty of solid reasons to integrate props into your yoga practice. If you're dealing with movement restrictions, such as muscle imbalances or contracture, props make it easy to move into an asana correctly. Props provide the flexibility for personalized modifications, allowing the poses to be adapted gradually to your specific ability over time. This, in turn, helps avoid frustrating situations like "I can't quite reach the floor with my hands in the Forward Bend," as yoga blocks or straps offer valuable support during the preparation phase for the pose.

1   B.K.S Iyengar, (1966). *Light on Yoga*, O.W. Barth Verlag

Props can also assist you to perceive specific areas of the body more distinctly, allowing you to grasp the essence of a pose. In this way, you can experience the pose holistically. As an experienced practitioner, the deliberate use of props enables you to refine and deepen your practice. Props allow you to hold a pose much longer, thereby experiencing deeper aspects of the practice. There are numerous other compelling reasons for incorporating props.

However, in certain situations, there are some arguments against integrating props into the practice. A prop always directs attention outward for a while. This can happen in very perception-oriented sessions where the focus is on energy flow. In a flow yoga class, the use of straps or blocks can be obstructive or simply take up too much time, thus interrupting the flow.

Regardless, an experienced and well-prepared yoga teacher knows the challenges and navigates them skillfully, incorporating these considerations into the planning process from the outset.

You've got a fantastic and highly successful book in your hands that will offer valuable inspiration for both your class preparation and your practice. In her book, Sara Lyn provides numerous variations and inspirations for both yoga teachers and individual practitioners. I had the honor of remotely accompanying the entire creation process of this work, and I wholeheartedly recommend it to my students, participants, and you.

–Martina Mittag
Author of *Hatha Yoga* (2019)

1
INTRODUCTION

After teaching yoga for eight years in various settings and working with people of diverse backgrounds and conditions, I found myself reflecting on what additional value another practice book could bring to the already expansive yoga world.

When I peruse my book collection, I mostly come across somewhat awkwardly translated literature, which I picked up during my time in India, where I completed my 200- and 300-hour training in Hatha, Ashtanga, and Vinyasa Yoga during a three-year period there. Along with my formal training, it was crucial for me to experience the spirit of yoga culture authentically.

So, my yoga journey didn't begin with a charismatic teacher who convinced me of yoga's physical benefits and values through a sequence of poses and a motivating soundtrack, as is often the case in Western studios today. Against the backdrop of my seventeen-year ballet career, Pilates initially transitioned me from the stage to the mat.

This workout devised by Joseph Hubert Pilates over a century ago primarily concentrates on strengthening the core. It employs a unique breathing technique to engage the deep muscles of the "Powerhouse," the core. Many dynamic Pilates exercises are inspired by yoga and are frequently used in rehabilitation sports and physiotherapy to support joints and enhance the function of restricted body parts.

Props such as balls, TheraBands, and fascia rollers are incorporated to ease the activation of deep muscles, amplify the impact of exercises, and fine-tune pelvic alignment. Despite my dedicated work as a Pilates instructor in fitness studios and sports clubs, I eventually felt the need for a different level of depth beyond what the physical workout provided.

How I Discovered Yoga

During my initial eight-month journey through Asia, a treat I gave myself after completing my bachelor's degree, my constant companion, alongside the exercise mat, was my first yoga book. It wasn't a widely recognized piece but a straightforward one that somehow ended up in my hands by chance. This unassuming book introduced me to the fundamental yoga poses of *Hatha Yoga*, a yoga form that acknowledges the physical benefits rooted in ancient philosophy.

Each morning, I dedicated about two hours to practicing the poses illustrated in the book. It quickly became apparent that, beyond the physical challenge, my mind was also undergoing a noticeable sharpening. Meditation and final relaxation were integral components of the fixed sequence in my morning routine, offering me a profound sense of inner focus. Yoga became a crucial anchor for me in my mid-twenties, being far from the familiar comforts of home.

After returning from my long journey, it became apparent that my next flight was destined for India. My eagerness to deepen my understanding of yoga led me to South India, specifically Goa, where I immersed myself in a four-week intensive training course. During this time, I delved into yoga teaching methodologies and embraced the minimalist lifestyle synonymous with being a yogi.

Back in the bustling city of Hamburg, I wasted no time and began teaching as much as possible. Passing on the wisdom of yoga and my insights into the connection between body and mind became my passion and calling. Eight years down the road, it remains the driving force behind the creation of this book.

"Yoga is the journey back to ourselves."

Since childhood and throughout my school days, books have held a unique sway over me. The conveyance of knowledge through words and illustrations is a valuable medium for universally sharing content.

Hence, this is precisely the approach I envisioned when crafting this work: presenting my insights on applying yoga postures alongside props in a simple and precise manner, making it a timeless piece for both yoga practitioners and teachers. I firmly believe that we are all simultaneously students and teachers.

"We are all equally students and teachers."

Purpose of the Book

Yoga serves as a path to heightened physical and mental awareness. If we can all acknowledge our state of mind and state of health, it can profoundly impact our physical and psychological health. Everyone should be able to embark on this journey, regardless of age, physical limitations, or external circumstances.

My intention is to meet each individual where they are in their practice and to guide them on their unique yoga path.

"Yoga is a path to greater physical and mental awareness."

To be open to the experiences along the way, the flexibility of the mind is more important than the body's flexibility. In Hatha Yoga, the physical body is used to access the spiritual core.

Originally, yoga poses were crafted to prepare the hips and spine for meditation. The body is regarded as the temple of the soul, necessitating maintenance in a pure and healthy state for ongoing growth. According to yoga, true mental repose and higher development are attainable only through meditation.

Achieving this requires mental focus cultivated through breath and a healthy, pain-free body. This book aims to make the yoga postures from Hatha Yoga accessible to everyone, contributing to a carefree life, whether in a spiritual or purely everyday consciousness.

"Mental flexibility is more important than the flexibility of the body."

2
YOGA
PHILOSOPHY

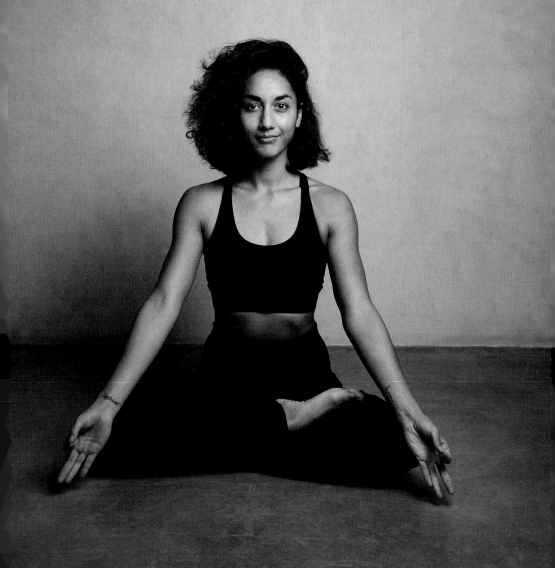

Yoga means *unity*. Only when body and mind are in sync do we grasp our true selves, free from the influences of matter, thoughts, and emotions. The yoga path instructs us to surmount the obstacles that divert us from self-realization and manifest in physical and mental imbalance.

Around 2,000 years ago, Patanjali, a significant trailblazer in yoga, documented his insights. In his book, *Yoga Sutras of Patanjali*, he introduced the eight-fold path of Ashtanga Yoga, which remains a global benchmark guide for yoga teachers and students.

The initial two stages of Patanjali's yogic journey are considered a moral code and general behaviors in how we deal with ourselves and others. The *Yamas* and *Niyamas* lay the groundwork for spiritual development on our life journeys.

Patanjali advocates for a non-violent, truthful, and clean way of life to progress to the subsequent stages of the yoga path. This path comprises *Asana* (yoga poses), *Pranayama* (breath control), *Pratyahara* (withdrawal of the senses), *Dharana* (concentration), *Dhyana* (meditation), and ultimately *Samadhi* (enlightenment).

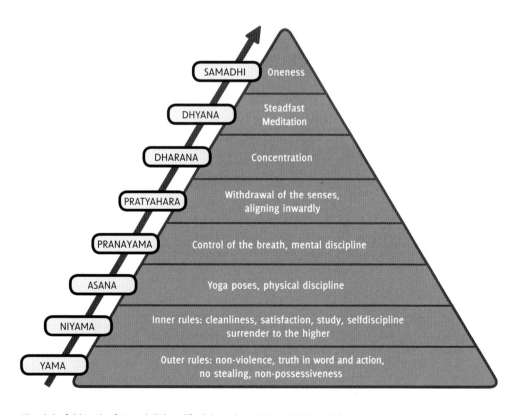

The eight-fold path of Patanjali (modified, based on Mittag, 2018, p.35)

In the concluding chapter of the Yoga Sutras, Patanjali delves into *Vyadhi* (physical ailments) that manifest on a psychological and emotional level. Even today, mitigating physical discomfort remains the primary motivation for practicing yoga in the Western world. However, the yogi's mental well-being can also experience improvement.

The autonomic nervous system, responsible for regulating unconscious bodily functions like relaxation and stress, is activated by the combination of conscious breathing and movement in yoga. With this blend, yoga exerts a more significant impact on the interplay of body and mind than most sports.

Recent research indicates that nerve structures are adaptable, and through movement and meditation practices, new connections can be established in the nervous system, overriding destructive activation patterns. This ability, known as *neuroplasticity*, is honed in yoga through meditation and mindfulness exercises.

By consciously recognizing our thoughts, movement, and action patterns, we can either maintain or enhance constructive aspects and, when necessary, discard or reshape others.

"The body is the temple of our souls."

—B.K.S Iyengar

On the yoga mat, the practitioner delves into conscious self-care, carving out a space to liberate themselves from external concerns, emotional fears, or economic factors that impose stress on the system. Although yoga can't control external events, it replenishes depleted energy reserves and empowers practitioners to radiate positive energy outward.

Good *karma* (good actions) is cultivated and shared in this manner. The circle completes as a reminder of the realization that everything is interconnected. This interconnectedness is evident in the etymology: yoga, derived from Sanskrit, roughly translates to *unity*.

Yoga Anatomy—the Koshas

The yogic anatomy breaks down the human body into five layers, or sheaths, called the *Koshas*. It is assumed that these layers envelop the spiritual core. Yoga asanas primarily target the outermost layer, *Annamaya Kosha* (food sheath).

By regulating the breath in Pranayama, we can stimulate Pranayama Kosha (vital sheath) and, through meditation, the mental sheath—*Manomaya Kosha*. The fourth sheath, *Vijnanamaya Kosha* (intellectual sheath), is influenced through engagement with spiritual scriptures and ultimately leads to the realization of *Anandamaya Kosha*—the blissful sheath.

If the yogi successfully penetrates all sheaths through persistent practice, the different levels converge, resulting in a sense of unity. In this context, asanas can serve as the initial step from body to soul consciousness on the yoga path.

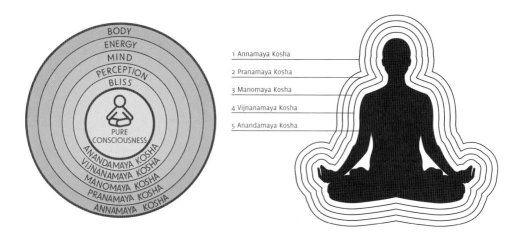

The Kosha model and the five sheaths

Prana and Chakras

The objective of Hatha Yoga is to harness the body for spiritual development. The yoga poses we assume on the mat aim to maintain strength and flexibility in the muscles and joints. Only by sustaining a healthy body can one fully dedicate oneself to spiritual growth without physical discomfort.

Prana, the life energy, can flow freely when physical blockages are released and the body is relaxed. This physical well-being can also guide us toward connecting with the higher self as we concentrate on the breath in meditation and enter a state of mental focus.

The central point is the spine. According to yogic anatomy, the seven main energy centers, known as *Chakras*, extend along the body's center. It is particularly crucial to keep the spine upright during meditation to release blockages in the chakras and supply them with Prana.

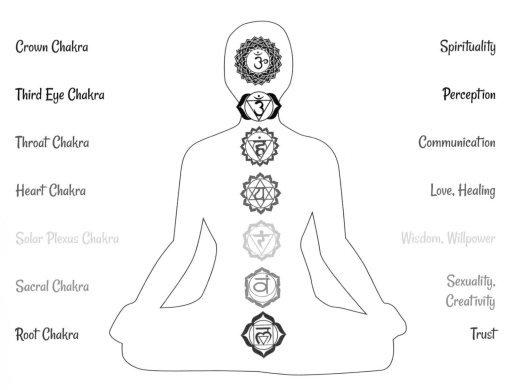

Crown Chakra	Spirituality
Third Eye Chakra	Perception
Throat Chakra	Communication
Heart Chakra	Love, Healing
Solar Plexus Chakra	Wisdom, Willpower
Sacral Chakra	Sexuality, Creativity
Root Chakra	Trust

The seven energy centers: the Chakras

Anyone who has spent an extended period in a seated meditation knows how challenging it is to keep the spine upright. In addition to strengthening the deep core muscles, Hatha Yoga aims to open the hips, allowing a yogi's body to remain relaxed even during prolonged meditation.

Targeted asanas focusing on specific body regions can be assumed alongside meditation to reach different chakras. Hip openers automatically stimulate the two lowest chakras: the *Root and Sacral Chakras*, representing our basic trust, as well as reproduction, sensuality, and creative power.

Twists target the fiery *Solar Plexus Chakra* in our body's center—our powerhouse needed for willpower, discipline, and transformation.

Backbends, however, pave the way to the *Heart and Throat Chakras*, the centers for love, compassion, and communication. Standing Forward Bends and inversions, such as headstands, shift attention to the two upper chakras—the *Third Eye* and the *Crown Chakra*—opening the gateway to oneself and cosmic consciousness.

As seen in classic Sun Salutations, the alternation between Forward and Backward Bends promotes spinal flexibility and positively influences the harmonious interplay of all chakras.

3
YOGA
Anatomy

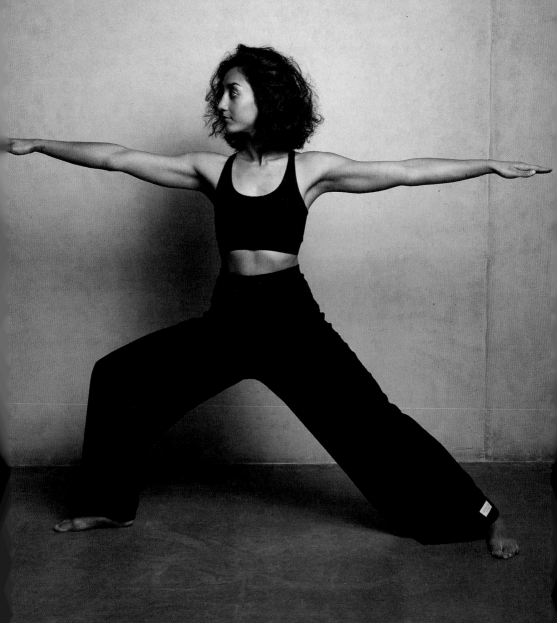

Medical Anatomy in Hatha Yoga

Hip Openers

The hip joint comprises the thigh bone and the corresponding pelvic socket on the same side, forming a ball-and-socket joint where the head of the thigh bone interacts with the hip socket of the pelvis. This spherical structure allows for a wide range of movement in the thigh bone, enabling us to move our legs in all directions.

Crucial for hip movement is a group of muscles collectively known as the **hip flexor muscles**. The main hip flexor, the *iliopsoas* (often abbreviated as psoas), connects the lower extremities to the lumbar spine, facilitating straightening through pelvic movement while sitting, standing, and walking.

The psoas is strengthened and stretched in standing yoga poses like Warriors I–III. Passive hip openers, such as the Reclining Butterfly (p.160) or Bridge Pose (p.104), aim to stretch the thigh and hip muscles.

The psoas has a direct connection to the diaphragm through its fascial structure. When stressed or experiencing shallow breathing, the hip muscles can tense up. It's no coincidence that the hips are considered the physical manifestation of our emotions in yoga. In Yin Yoga, prolonged, deep stretches can assist in releasing emotional blockages in this area.

A more minor muscle central to many yoga poses is the *piriformis*. If this muscle is shortened, it can cause discomfort along the sciatic nerve just below it. Numerous deep hip openers target this pear-shaped muscle beneath the buttocks and can provide relief from lower back pain.

Hip opening is not just about flexibility; it also contributes to maintaining an upright pelvis posture. Well-rounded training of the hip and leg muscles aids in centering the hip joint. A pelvis tilted forward or backward stresses the intervertebral discs and should be corrected through conscious alignment in yoga poses.

The use of yoga blocks in standing asanas encourages upright alignment and facilitates deep hip-opening poses, especially when there's a limited range of motion in the hip joints.

While the hip joint is typically one of the most mobile in the body, significant anatomical differences exist from one skeleton to another. Consequently, regardless of the amount of practice, not everyone may be able to assume certain yoga poses, like the Lotus pose. The incorporation of props, however, can make a substantial difference for individuals with less flexible hips.

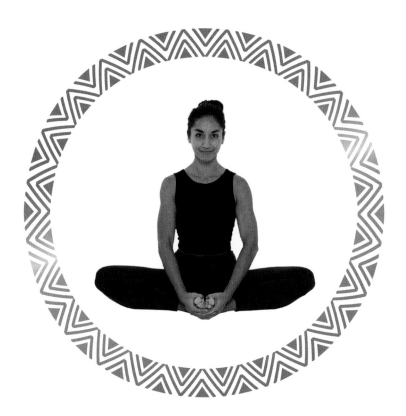

Forward Bends

In general, Forward Bends in yoga elongate the back of the body. Standing Forward Bends, like *Uttanasana* (p. 42), have an opening effect on the entire posterior fascial chain, from the soles of the feet to the back of the head. On the other hand, seated Forward Bends focus more on stretching the back and possibly the back of the legs. Forward Bends also calm the autonomic nervous system, helping us truly quiet the mind.

Forward Bends are often viewed as a benchmark for physical flexibility. From a mental standpoint, they teach us patience and to embrace our physical limitations. Calm breathing, especially a deepened exhalation, holds particular significance here because, according to yoga philosophy, it allows for the physical and mental release of old structures. Over time, this takes us deeper into the pose and a state of mental tranquility.

In the withdrawal from the Forward Bend, we can connect with ourselves without being distracted by external influences. The deeper the Forward Bend, the more profound the effect on the entire system.

When the thighs and abdomen touch, as in *Paschimottanasana* (p. 137), the movement of the breath and the additional counterpressure from the outside intensely stimulate the abdominal organs, positively influencing digestion.

Props also enable experiencing the holistic benefits of Forward Bends, even with limited mobility.

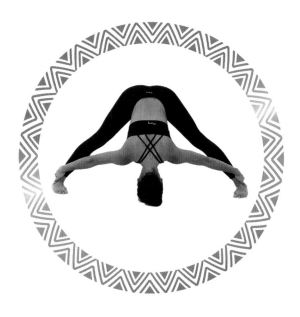

Backbends

In contrast to Forward Bends, Backbends are acknowledged as stimulators of the sympathetic nervous system, the branch of the autonomic nervous system responsible for physical performance and triggered in the *fight-or-flight mode*. They carry a revitalizing effect on the mind, countering lethargy, depressive moods, and fatigue.

These poses contribute to strengthening back muscles, imparting a feeling of physical strength. The extension of the front of the body opens the chest and respiratory spaces, enhancing oxygen supply to the organs, particularly benefiting lung and heart muscle function. Consistent and mindful practice of Backbends enhances overall flexibility in the torso.

Engaging in deep Backbends like *Urdhva Dhanurasana*—Wheel Pose (p. 107) demands precise execution and careful preparation. For instance, if there's a lack of shoulder strength, yoga blocks can serve as valuable support. Once the mental challenge of entering the posture is overcome, the effects become immediately noticeable.

Regrettably, many individuals develop an excessively rounded upper spine (hyperkyphosis) due to sedentary habits and prolonged desk posture. The use of smartphones has even led young people to adopt misalignments that can be corrected through the practice of Backbends.

The deep breath facilitated by the *heart openers* instills a sense of freedom in the system. It propels us away from feelings of confinement, opening us up to the world, free from fears and constraints.

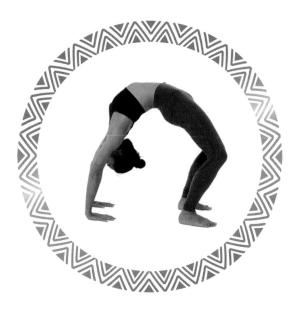

Twisting Poses

The back is prepared for intense twists through preceding movements in the spine, such as Forward and Backward Bends. Depending on the intensity of the asana, twists have a liberating effect: blockages in the thoracic spine can be alleviated in passive postures, like *Jathara Parivartanasana* (p. 168), proving very soothing for back pain. Meanwhile, active twists, originating more from the body's center, collaborate with breathing to stimulate the detoxification function of digestive organs.

Deepening the breath in twisting poses operates like a massage for internal organs (for example, the liver on the right side) and triggers increased blood circulation upon releasing the corresponding pose. This results in a sensation of physical and mental clarity, which is why yoga twists are practiced for vitality and cleansing of the entire system.

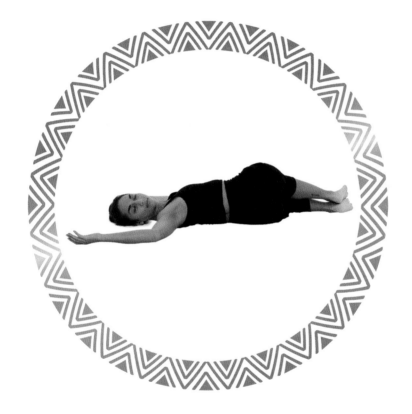

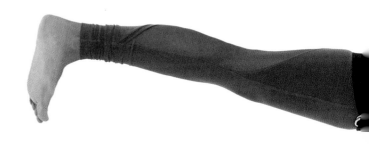

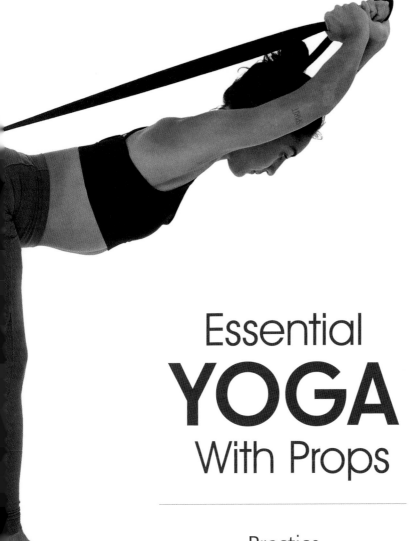

Essential
YOGA
With Props

Practice

"Yoga strengthens the connection between the mental and physical levels, thus creating a sense of inner and outer balance. When we achieve these alignments, every cell and fiber of our body is in perfect harmony."

–B.K.S Iyengar

A pioneer in incorporating props into yoga was **B.K.S. Iyengar** (1918–2014). Driven by poverty and physical ailments, the young Iyengar accepted an invitation from his brother-in-law to be trained in his yoga school.

In the 1930s, in the southern Indian city of Mysore, the top students of the legendary guru Krishnamarcharya underwent training to perfect their yoga asanas. Pose, discipline, and perseverance defined his students, profoundly shaping the yoga practice for generations.

Iyengar recognized the potential harm that incorrectly performed or unprepared asanas could inflict on the body and mind. He dedicated his life to thoroughly studying yoga postures and developing a method that enabled everyone to experience the benefits of Hatha Yoga.

His vision aimed to provide each student, per their abilities, the opportunity to achieve a unified harmony without the risk of misalignments or injuries. Under his guidance, yoga props like wooden blocks, straps, and ropes were introduced.

The use of props in this book

Many yogic theories about the human body are now considered outdated and have limited applicability to the modern body. This book does not intend to force the body into a posture, which is not in harmony with its anatomy. The standard props in yoga classes are meant for precise alignment and the most effective yoga practice.

The selection of postures and their variations with props is rooted in my extensive experience as a yoga teacher, aiming to offer optimistic inspiration for fellow teachers and provide newcomers with the opportunity to tailor their yoga practice to their bodies.

In collaboration with physiotherapist Maike Lüders and osteopath, yoga, and movement teacher, as well as physiotherapist Cornelius Feist, we delved into crucial insights into the holistic anatomy of the human body. This encompasses muscles, fascia, joints, as well as the nervous system and organs.

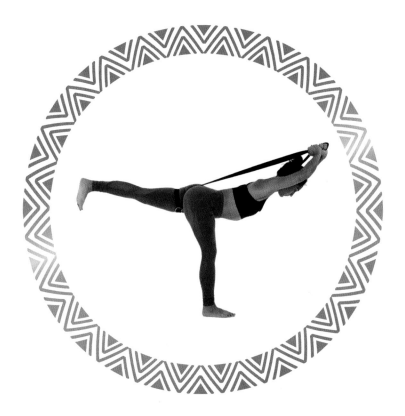

The yoga block

The yoga block has been a staple in modern yoga practice for several decades. Initially crafted from wood, it served as a sturdy aid for refining and adjusting standing postures during the era of B.K.S. Iyengar. It proves especially beneficial for newcomers or individuals with limited mobility.

For instance, a yoga block can support the hand on the floor during poses like *Parshvakonasana*—Extended Side Angle Pose or *Trikonasana*—Triangle Pose (p. 72). In seated Forward Bends, it often comes into play for enhancing hip stretches or engaging deep core muscles, as seen in *Navasana*—Boat Pose (p. 101).

Newer yoga forms like Power or Core Yoga focus on strengthening the deep abdominal muscles. Here, the block is an activating aid for the pelvic floor and the *transversus abdominis* muscle, for example, when the block is clamped between the thighs and held there by muscle activity.

This technique can also be transferred to other postures, such as *Utkatasana* (Chair Pose), to focus on the body's center. The yoga block can also be used as an additional weight for hands or legs in strength training.

In addition to modification and activation, the block is helpful in Yin Yoga for relaxation in postures. In Yin Yoga, more or less passive yoga postures are held for 3-5 minutes. The block can serve as support for the body to allow an elevated position of the chest. This way, the practitioner can fully hold the pose and focus entirely on the breath without having to concentrate on activating muscles and joints.

There are now yoga blocks made of foam that may be suitable for specific purposes due to their light and soft material. However, for the exercises in this book, I recommend a cork yoga block—a sustainable natural material that is not as hard and heavy as wood but more robust than a foam block.

The yoga strap

The yoga strap is another widely embraced prop, suitable for standing, seated, or reclining poses. When dealing with rigid shoulders, it proves invaluable for opening up the chest. In specific poses, particularly for individuals with short arms or contracted chest muscles, integrating a strap can make a big difference.

While holding the strap, the practitioner must sustain consistent muscle tension. This facilitates an active stretch as the muscles under tension undergo strengthening and simultaneous lengthening. This dual effect contributes to stretching and strengthening muscles near the joints.

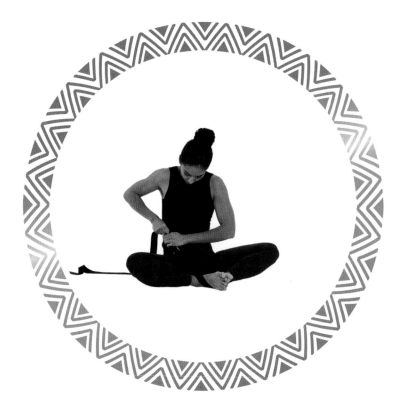

Especially when guiding sequences involving the strap, offering clear instructions to students about the appropriate buckle placement in each posture proves helpful.

The yoga bolster

The yoga bolster is a key support tool primarily used in passive yoga poses. It is most useful in Yin or Restorative Yoga, where practitioners hold relaxed yoga poses for extended durations ranging from 5 to 20 minutes. The cylindrical cushion is strategically deployed to minimize the muscular effort required.

This proves incredibly soothing for the spine, whether in the context of Backbends, such as the Reclining Butterfly (p. 160) or Forward Bends, as seen in the Wide-Angle Seated Forward Bend (p. 127).

The goal is to distribute the entire body weight onto the bolster without compromising its form. Most bolsters are filled with spelt or kapok. A standard size of 60 x 30 x 15 centimeters (23 x 12 x 5 in) caters to a broad spectrum of practitioners, irrespective of body size.

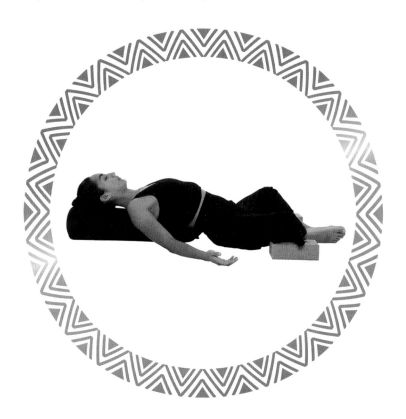

4
STRENGTH
& Alignment

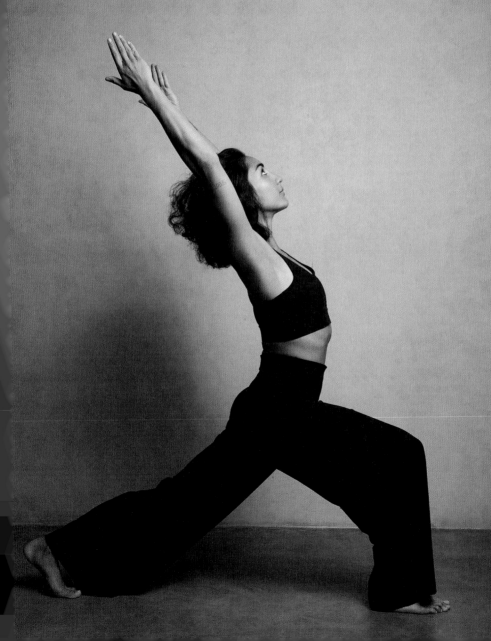

Tadasana—Mountain Pose

Tada = Mountain

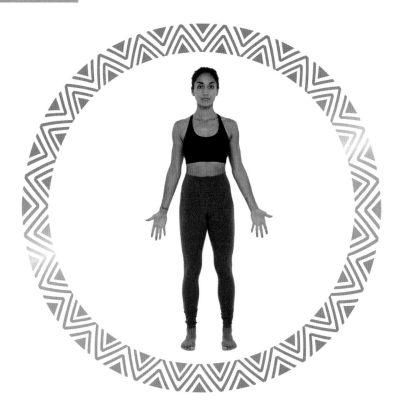

Tadasana, the Mountain Pose, is the foundation for all standing poses in Hatha Yoga. Even B.K.S Iyengar knew how demanding an upright and healthy posture is and referred to it as "the art of flawless standing."

Depending on the Tradition, there are various interpretations of *Tadasana*. In the Sun Salutation sequence, the upright stance is also referred to as *Samasthithi*, which translates to "Steadiness." In all its variations, this asana aims to improve posture.

By assuming the posture of a mountain, we build bodily tension and engage the muscles from head to toe. The mindfulness required in establishing the pose also demands our mental focus. It serves as the perfect preparation for practicing sequences of standing asanas.

Tadasana with a block

Alignment of the feet

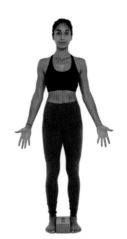

1. Place the yoga block between the insides of your feet.

2. Activate your feet by lifting the balls of the feet while keeping the toes firmly on the ground.

3. Lift the heels and extend them backward before firmly grounding the outer edge of the foot on the mat. The heel bone should feel wide as a result. The ankle bones are aligned precisely parallel to each other.

Notice the difference when you remove the block from between your feet. The foot's arch should still be lifted and the sole firmly grounded.

The feet are the foundation of the posture. Their alignment significantly affects the alignment of the knees, hips, and spine. The block aids in heightening your awareness of your feet in an upright stance and guides you in activating the arches.

Alignment of the knees

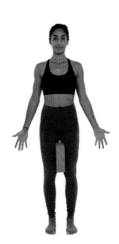

1. Place the yoga block between the insides of your knees.

2. Extend your legs and activate the thigh muscles to lift the kneecaps upward. Press the insides of your knees into the block. Keep the gluteal muscles relaxed.

The resistance of the block activates the knees and helps focus on engaging your thigh muscles. This is particularly helpful for individuals with bowlegs or knock-knees to enhance posture and protect the knees.

Alignment of the pelvis

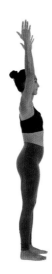 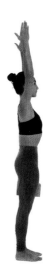

1.   Place the yoga block between your thighs.

2.   Press the insides of your thighs against the block. Bring your feet closer together so the pressure is evenly distributed on both sides.

3.   Roll the insides of your thighs inward as if you were trying to move the block backward.

4.   At the same time, activate your gluteal muscles and move your tailbone forward as if you were trying to push the block forward.

5.   Slide the front of your thighs backward.

Stay in this pose for several deep breaths.

The activation of the leg muscles aims at the inner rotation of the thighs. This provides better stability for the posture and enables proper pelvis alignment.

Tadasana with a strap

Relief of the pelvis/sacroiliac joints

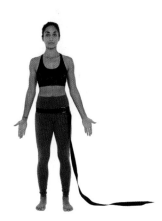 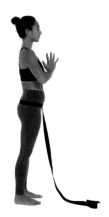

1. Place the strap around the middle part of your pelvis.

2. Bend your knees slightly and tighten the strap, ensuring it's snug around the outside of the pelvic bones and noticeable in the center of the sacrum.

Stay in this pose for several deep breaths.

By applying gentle pressure on the pelvic bones, the strap sensitizes awareness of the hips. This especially benefits those with hip issues and relieves the sacroiliac joint.

Alignment of the shoulders/chest opening

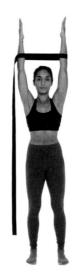 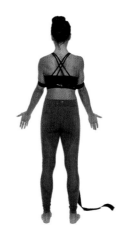

1. Place the strap around the forearms at shoulder width.

2. Lift the sternum and push the arms down, extending the fingertips toward the mat.

3. Push the outer sides of your forearms into the strap as if trying to widen it sideways.

4. Turn the palms forward and the thumbs further outward.

Stay in this pose for several deep breaths. Notice how the sternum lifts higher with each breath, creating space within the sides of the body. As you exhale, let the shoulders sink lower. The area between the shoulder blades relaxes.

To emphasize the activity of the upper arms, you can raise the arms straight overhead. The distance between the shoulders and ears should remain the same.

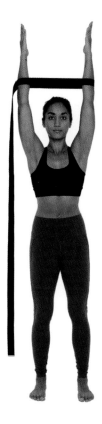

The activation of the arms against the resistance of the strap brings the shoulders outward and the shoulder blades closer together. This results in chest opening, positively impacting breathing and widening the heart space.

Uttanasana—Standing Forward Bend

Uttana = stretch

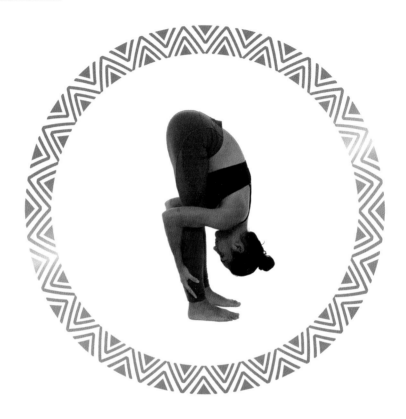

Uttanasana, the standing Forward Bend, is also known as the intense forward stretch. By bending the torso over the stretched legs, the entire back of the body is stretched, especially the back of the legs.

The legs and core muscles should be especially activated to stabilize the body in the inversion. The head-down position slows down the heartbeat, and the body's stress level can be reduced.

Forward Bends always involve an introverted posture, allowing the release of thoughts and mental heaviness. This calming effect on the nervous system is particularly beneficial for exhaustion caused by stress, anxiety, or depression.

Uttanasana with two blocks

Activation of the back of the legs/pelvic alignment

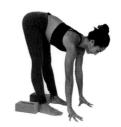

1. Stand with your back against a wall. Place two flat blocks vertically between your heels and the wall. The feet are hip width apart.

2. Come forward with a straight back into *Ardha Uttanasana*—the Half-Forward Bend.

3. Put your hand on your hips and roll the buttocks up and back so you can firmly push the sit bones into the wall.

4. Bring your fingertips to the mat, inhale, and with a long spine, bend over the stretched legs.

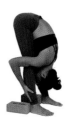

5. Exhale and relax the torso downward toward your thighs.

Stay in this pose for several deep breaths. With each exhale, let yourself sink deeper into the stretch.

The support of the wall and the blocks helps maintain the straight alignment of the pelvis. The hips are often imbalanced and not properly aligned, which is challenging to correct in free space. This alignment prevents the habit of a tilted pelvic posture and enhances the stretch of the backs of the legs.

Uttanasana with two blocks and a strap

Pelvic alignment/activation of the back of the legs

1. Step into the loop of the strap with both feet. Hold the outer edges of the strap in both hands.

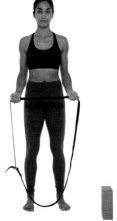

2. Place both feet on the front part of the strap. Bend forward from the hips and place the back part of the strap on the tailbone. Ensure the buckle of the strap is within reach.

3. Bend both knees gently and tighten the strap to encircle your pelvis firmly.

4. Slowly lift the buttocks and straighten the legs against the resistance of the strap. If you don't feel enough support, change the width of the strap.

5. Slide the outer sides of your thighs into the strap to keep it taut. Lift the kneecaps and the inner sides of your ankles gently.

6. Place your hands on two vertically upright blocks. The blocks should be directly under your shoulders.

7. Inhale and lengthen the spine forward from the hips into *Ardha Uttanasana*—the Half-Forward Bend.

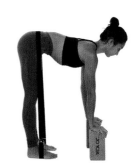

8. As you exhale, bring your hands down to the mat and ease into *Uttanasana*—the complete Forward Bend. It's okay to bend both knees, slightly relieving tension in the strap. Keep the lower back elongated, letting the upper body gently descend onto the thighs.

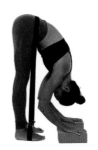

Stay in this pose for several deep breaths. Sink deeper into the Forward Bend with each exhale.

The strap keeps the pelvis in a snug alignment with the legs, enabling the lumbar spine to extend backward. This actively stretches the back of the legs, ensuring the lower back maintains its length before the bend. The stabilization of the hips provides relief to the lower back.

Uttanasana variation with a block

Shoulder stretch/chest opening

1. Hold a block between your hands behind your back. Press the palms into the block to activate the front shoulder and chest muscles.

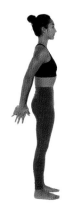

2. Inhale, roll your shoulders back, away from your ears, and extend your arms to open your chest even further.

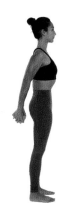

3. Breathe out and bend forward over the stretched legs into *Uttanasana*.

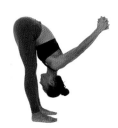

Stay in this pose for a few deep breaths. Notice how your chest expands more with each inhale. Let yourself gradually sink deeper into the Forward Bend with each exhale. Lower the block back to your buttocks slowly and rise with a long back.

This variation of Uttanasana helps people with stiff shoulders and shortened chest muscles to open the chest further. This deepens the breath and relaxes the neck muscles.

Anjaneyasana—Low Crescent Lunge

Anjaneya = half moon

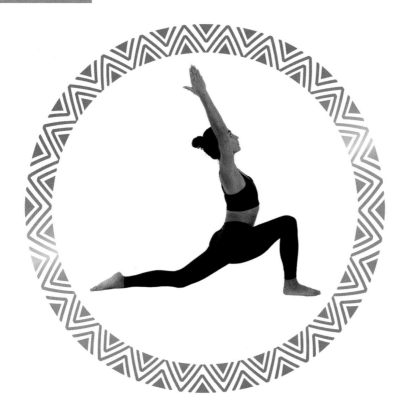

The Low Crescent Lunge is based on the flexibility of the monkey god *Hanuman*, also known as *Anjaneya*, who, according to Hindu mythology, is famous for his wide jumps.

This deep lunge not only elongates the hip muscles, fostering flexibility for activities like jumping or running, but also relieves the lower back by stretching the hip flexor *(iliopsoas)* originating from the lumbar spine. Furthermore, the expansive Backbend characteristic of this pose serves to open up the chest.

In its complete manifestation, *Anjaneyasana* is both a hip and heart opener, directly influencing the sacral and heart chakras. If dealing with acute lower back concerns, it's crucial to pay special attention to the precise execution and alignment of the pelvis in this posture.

Anjaneyasana with two blocks

Pelvic alignment

1. Place two blocks upright at the front of the mat.

2. Move into a deep Forward Bend and place your hands on the blocks.

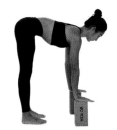

3. Step the right leg back, taking a large stride with the left leg.

4. Lower the knee to the mat.

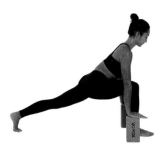

5. Move the blocks further back, aligning them directly under the shoulders. Place the top of the back foot on the mat. Inhale, lift the chest. Exhale and sink deeper into the pelvis.

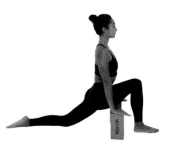

Keep the upper body upright as you sink deeper into the hips. Relax the back of the shoulder blades.

Stay in this pose for several deep breaths. With each inhalation, the front of the body opens. With each exhalation, let the pelvis sink deeper.

The elevation through the blocks aids in aligning the torso over the pelvis, creating more length in the hip and abdominal muscles leading to an overall extension of the front body. Specifically, the quadriceps and the iliopsoas muscle are stretched.

Alanasana—High Lunge

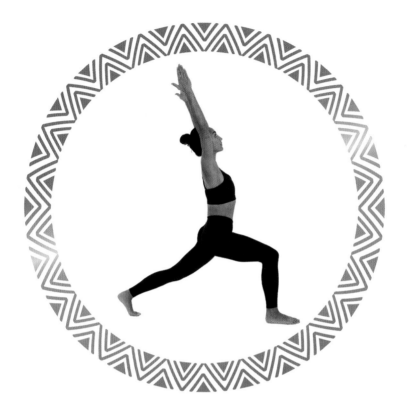

Alanasana represents an advanced take on *Anjaneyasana*, frequently adopted as a variation of *Warrior I* (p. 66). The key distinction lies in pointing the back toes to elevate the foot, ensuring a straight alignment of the pelvis, and enhancing the stretch of the hip flexor.

Alanasana with a strap

Shoulder Strengthening

1. Begin by holding a strap at shoulder width in front of the chest. Step into a wide lunge with both legs bent, ensuring the back toes are pointed and the hip is closed.

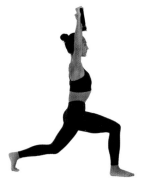

2. Inhale as you lift the strap overhead, fully extending the arms while keeping the strap taut.

3. Powerfully extend the back leg from the hip flexor. Maintaining a long upper body, gently lean back for a stretch of your front body.

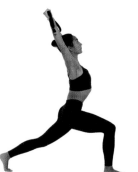

Stay in this pose for several deep breaths. Feel the chest expand with each inhalation, and pull the strap firmly with each exhalation. Lower the arms slowly, then switch sides.

This variation effectively strengthens the shoulder muscles by working against the resistance of the strap. Simultaneously, the upper part of the chest muscles is actively stretched. It is beneficial for mobilizing the thoracic spine and shoulder joints and is particularly effective for those with stiff shoulders.

Activation of the upper arms

1. Turn the strap into a shoulder-width loop.

2. Step into a wide lunge with the back toes pointed and the hips closed.

3. Place your forearms into the strap.

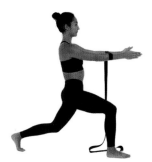

4. As you inhale, raise the strap overhead, fully extending the arms.

5. Actively press the forearms against the inner sides of the strap. Bring the shoulder blades together and rotate the thumbs backward.

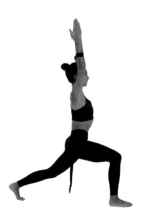

Hold this pose for several deep breaths. Lower the arms and switch sides.

In this variation, the upper arms are deliberately activated separately from the upper trapezius. This allows the shoulder girdle to descend, alleviating strain on the neck muscles.

Adho Mukha Svanasana—Downward Facing Dog

Adho = down, *Mukha* = face, *Svan* = dog

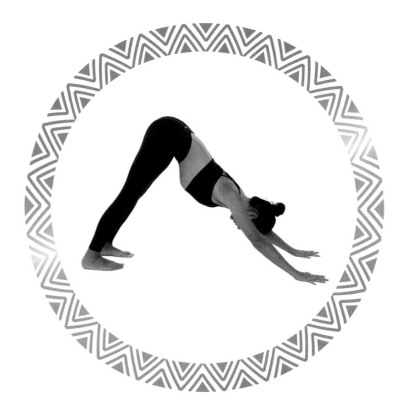

Downward Facing Dog is one of the most popular poses in Hatha Yoga and, as the name suggests, is inspired by the stretching movement of a dog. In its correct execution, the outer form of the asana resembles a triangle. The tailbone forms the highest point, akin to the summit of a mountain, which is why *Adho Mukha Svanasana* is also known as the *Mountain Pose* in other traditions.

Energetically, *Downward Facing Dog*, like all other inversion poses, has a cooling effect on the nervous system. Unlike classical Forward Bends, it is considered an activating asana. The entire back of the body is stretched, with particular emphasis on stretching the calves and upper thigh muscles while simultaneously strengthening the shoulders and arms.

Initially, the pose may seem challenging because it requires strength in the shoulders, arms, and upper back, and many people tend to have shortened leg muscles, making it difficult to straighten the legs. The use of props can assist in progressing toward a more comfortable pose.

Strengthening the fronts of the thighs/intensive stretch in the lower legs

1. Place two blocks flat against the wall.

2. Turn with your back to the wall, heels leaning against the blocks.

3. Come into the Forward Bend, walk the hands forward, and move into *Downward Facing Dog.*

4. Place the feet one in front of the other on the outer edges of the blocks.

5. Push the heels into the blocks until the toes lift and spread.

6. Extend the legs further.

7. Actively hold the legs in this pose for several breaths.

8. Return your feet to the mat, press the back soles firmly into the ground, and push the heels toward the outer edges of the blocks.

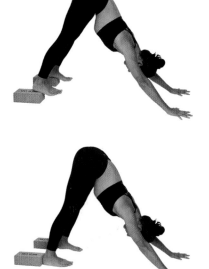

*This variation helps strengthen the thigh muscles in **Downward Facing Dog**. The spine can be extended further by shifting the weight onto the heels. The backs of the legs are intensely stretched, increasing the range of motion in the ankles.*

Adho Mukha Svanasana with blocks against the wall

Activation of the hands and forearms/centering of the shoulder joints/relief of the cervical spine

1. Place two flat blocks vertically, shoulder width apart, against a wall.

2. Place your palms on the blocks, with thumbs enclosing the inner sides of the blocks.

3. Walk the feet back into *Downward Facing Dog*.

4. Shift the weight forward until the shoulders are over the hands.

5. Slightly bend the arms and rotate the upper arms outward so that your elbows gently point to the sides.

6. Rotate the inner arms toward the shoulders.

7. Slowly begin to straighten the arms.

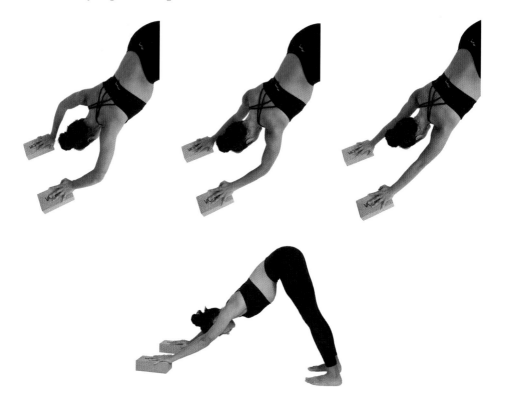

The lower part of the palms pushes against the block's lower edge. The fingers are widely spread and pointing upwards.

Stay in this pose for several deep breaths, and slowly come out of the pose by walking the feet toward the hands. Stay in a deep Forward Bend for a moment before straightening up.

Pushing into the blocks activates the fingers, hand arches, forearms, and shoulders. The correct alignment and activation of the arms in **Downward Facing Dog** *are crucial as they affect the movement of the shoulder blades.*

If the shoulder blades are moved toward the spine through the rotational movement of the arms, there is no pressure on the thoracic spine and head. Furthermore, arm strength helps prevent injury and misalignment in the shoulders. This variation is also suitable for people with shorter arms or significantly shortened backs of the legs to bring the heels closer to the ground.

Adho Mukha Svanasana with a blanket

Relief for the wrists

1. Fold a thin blanket or towel horizontally and place it at the front of the mat.

2. Come into *Downward Facing Dog* and place the lower part of the palms on the front edge of the blanket.

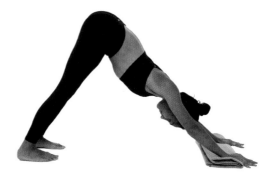

Elevating the hands relieves the wrists. This variation is particularly suitable for everyone experiencing wrist pain.

Adho Mukha Svanasana with a bolster

Relief of the cervical spine

1.   Place a bolster vertically at the front of the mat.

2.   Come into *Downward Facing Dog* and rest the forehead on the bolster.

3.   Stay in this pose for several deep breaths. Consciously deepen the exhale and feel the calming effect on the brain.

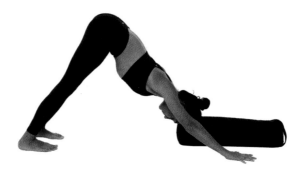

For many people, remaining in an inversion pose for an extended period may feel unfamiliar. The bolster supports the cervical spine and allows for a more profound relaxation in the pose.

Chaturanga Dandasana—Four-Limbed Staff

Chatur = four, *Anga* = limb, *Danda* = stick/staff

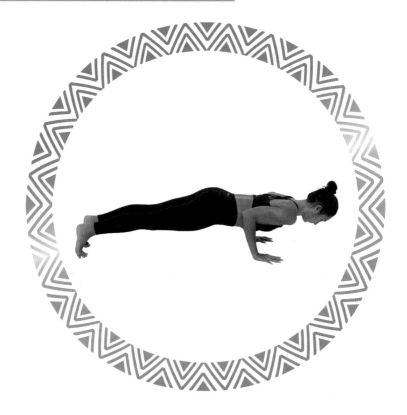

Chaturanga Dandasana, also known as Yoga Push-Up, is a potent pose that acts as a transition from *Downward Facing Dog* to a prone position.

The challenge lies in maintaining a right angle at the elbows, as the body weight is supported by the hands and feet, engaging the shoulders, arms, chest, and core muscles.

In dynamic transitions within Vinyasa Yoga,* the precision of the pose can often be compromised. Using yoga blocks to ensure the correct alignment becomes invaluable in preparing the body for such demanding poses.

* *Vinyasa Yoga = a contemporary and less static form of yoga that traces its roots back to traditional Ashtanga Yoga. Its dynamic sequence of yoga poses is practiced in harmony with the flow of the breath.*

Chaturanga Dandasana with a block

Activation of arm and core muscles

1. Lie on your stomach and position the block flat under the pelvis.

2. Bring your hands under the shoulders, keeping your thumbs close to the body.

3. Place your toes on the ground and activate the thigh and glute muscles.

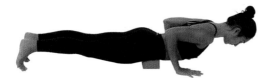

4. Roll the shoulder blades toward the spine and firmly press the hands into the ground.

5. Engage the core muscles and lift the pelvis off the block.

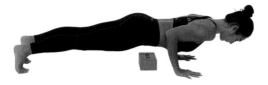

6. Lower yourself down, take a deep breath, and repeat the movement several times.

For most individuals, supporting the body weight on the arms can initially pose a challenge. Elevating the pelvis with the block diminishes the impact of gravity, making it easier to lift the body.

Chaturanga Dandasana with two blocks

Arm alignment

1. Place two upright blocks at the front of the mat.

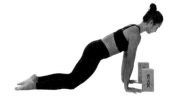

2. Come up onto your knees and position your hands in front of the blocks.

3. Bend the arms close to the body, allowing the shoulders to rest on the blocks.

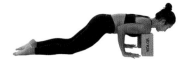

4. Place your toes on the ground, shift the heels back, and lift the knees off the mat. Engage the thigh and glute muscles while the navel draws inward and upward.

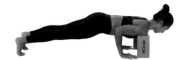

5. Hold this position for several deep breaths before lowering the knees back to the ground.

The blocks provide essential support to bear the body weight and enhance alignment in the pose. Many individuals have an imbalanced body posture when static, often stemming from unilateral movements in daily life. The blocks help identify potential asymmetries in the shoulders and assist in addressing them.

Urdhva Mukha Svanasana—Upward Facing Dog

Urdhva = upward, *Mukha* = face, *Svan* = dog

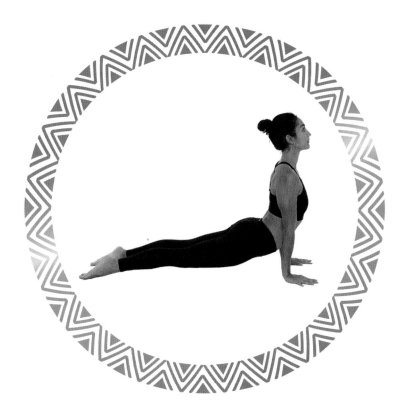

Urdhva Mukha Svanasana is an intense Backbend that demands significant strength in the shoulders and arms. *Upward Facing Dog* is used to complement *Downward Facing Dog* to elongate the front body in Vinyasa flows.

The chest opens much wider than in, for instance, *Bhujangasana* (Cobra Pose), which is often chosen as a more back-friendly alternative in Sun Salutations because the elbows stay bent and the thighs remain relaxed on the mat. This pose profoundly influences the abdomen, heart, and throat chakras when executed accurately.

Lifting the legs stretches the muscles in the thighs and hips and, more importantly, strengthens them. However, individuals with lower back or spine issues should refrain from practicing this Backbend.

Urdva Mukha Svanasana with two blocks

Support for the Backbend

1. Place two flat blocks vertically at the front of the mat.

2. Get into the tabletop position with your hands on the blocks under the shoulders.

3. Extend your legs backward, one at a time, moving into the Plank pose.

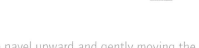

4. Engage the abdominal muscles by lifting the navel upward and gently moving the ribs toward the spine.

5. Place the tops of your feet down, one at a time, and lower the pelvis for Upward Facing Dog. The instep presses into the mat, and the knees are lifted off the mat.

6. Using your arm strength, push away from the blocks, lifting the chest forward.

7. Rotate the upper arms outward and draw the shoulder blades toward each other.

Stay in this pose for a few deep breaths.

The support of the hands on the blocks relieves the wrists, activating the shoulders. The elevation through the blocks intensifies the stretch in the groins, quadriceps, and abdominal region, allowing for a deeper stretch often lost during transitions in the Vinyasa flow.

Pincha Mayurasana—Forearm Balance

Pincha = feather, *Mayura* = peacock

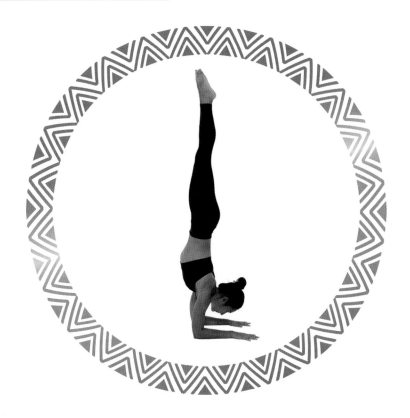

Forearm Balance is among the inversions that promote blood circulation, activating both the cardiovascular and the body's drainage system. This, in turn, positively impacts the musculoskeletal, digestive, nervous, and cardiovascular systems.

From a muscular perspective, the pose mainly involves the shoulders and arms, necessitating a flexible thoracic spine. Opening the heart space contributes positively to the heart chakra and fosters self-confidence on a mental level.

Pincha Mayurasana with a block and a strap (against the wall)

Shoulder girdle strengthening/arm alignment

1. Position a flat block horizontally against the wall.

2. Loop a yoga strap around the forearms, ensuring it's pulled tight to prevent slipping and maintain the arms aligned at shoulder width

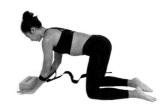

3. Kneel in front of the wall, focus your gaze on the yoga block, and place the forearms on it, with the knees under the hips, resembling the tabletop position.

4. Form an L-shape with the thumbs and index fingers around the corners of the block, and ensure the hands lie flat on the floor.

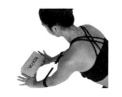

5. Press your elbows into the mat, actively push the forearms into the strap, and rotate the shoulder blades toward the spine to engage the shoulder girdle.

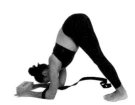

6. Rise onto the toes, lift the knees off the mat, and begin to extend the legs.

7. Walk the feet closer to the arms while keeping the shoulder position unchanged.

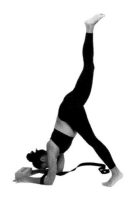

8.   Lift one leg and generate a gentle upward momentum. Bring the feet to the wall and balance slowly.

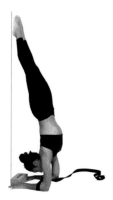

The arms serve as the foundation for the pose. The strap prevents the external rotation of the shoulders, ensuring the elbows stay in place and preserve the stability of the pose. The block is an additional arm alignment aid, offering extra stability to the shoulder girdle.

Virabhadrasana I—Warrior I

Vira = brave, *Bhadra* = gracious

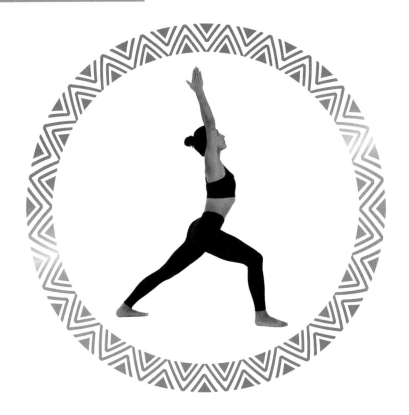

Virabhadra is the name of a warrior in Indian mythology, hence the standard reference to *Virabhadrasana* as Warrior Pose. The Warrior embodies qualities of steadfastness, serenity, and self-confidence.

The cornerstone of *Warrior I* lies in the foundation provided by the feet. The back foot is subtly turned outward, roughly 45 degrees, while the front foot points directly ahead. The front leg is bent in line with the ankle, demonstrating powerful engagement through the thigh muscles.

Maintaining a grounded back foot is essential for stretching the back leg. The foot's arch is raised, and the seamless transfer of strength from the foot to the thigh lends crucial support to the knee joint in this pose.

When the weight is evenly distributed on both legs, the pose benefits by establishing a connection from the back leg through the pelvis to the torso. This facilitates the stretching of the hip flexor, contributing to the intense extension of the spine.

Maintaining a straightly aligned pelvis poses the most significant challenge in this posture. Shortened muscles in the back leg can cause difficulty in lowering the heel.

As an alternative, *Alanasana*, the High Lunge (p. 49), is often practiced, keeping the toes of the back foot pointed.

Virabhadrasana I with a strap

Activation of the thigh/spinal stretch/chest opening

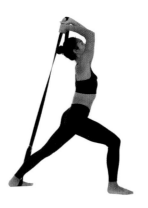

1. Begin by standing on one end of your mat. Create a small loop in the strap.

2. Place your left foot in the loop of the strap, holding the long end of the strap in your left hand.

3. Take a large step forward with your right foot, ensuring the left foot is turned slightly outward (about 45 degrees). Secure the back foot in the loop, with the front thigh rotating slightly inward and the back thigh rotating slightly outward.

4. Lift the arms straight up to the sides and reach with the right hand for the strap.

5. Hold the strap in both hands, ensuring your elbows point forward and up.

6.   Lengthen and lift the strap, feeling the spine straighten further and the chest opening.

7.   Press the outer edge of the back foot more firmly into the loop. By extending the strap, the thigh rotates further outward.

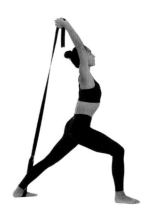

Remain in this pose for several deep breaths, then switch to the other side.

The strap activates the back thigh and supports its external rotation, which is necessary for pelvic stability. The spine is stretched out of the lifted and aligned pelvis by lengthening the yoga strap.

The strap connects all essential body parts in this pose, emphasizing the foundation of the back foot on the ground and the extension of the spine upward, allowing the chest to open more fully.

Alternatively, to emphasize the external rotation of the back thigh, the strap can be placed around the thigh. This also accentuates the straight alignment of the pelvis.

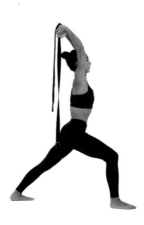

Virabhadrasana II—Warrior II

Vira = brave, *Bhadra* = gracious

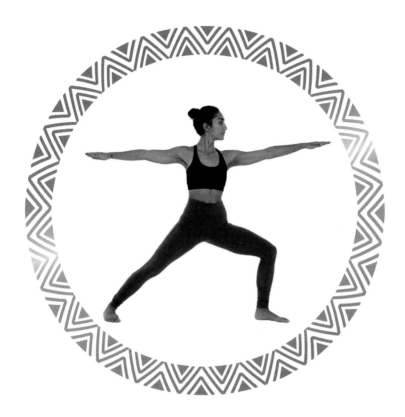

Warrior II is considered one of the most well-known standing poses in Hatha Yoga, symbolizing balance and steadfastness. The challenge lies in maintaining a vertical alignment of the spine over the pelvis without shifting too much weight into the bent front leg.

Steadfastness, on a physical level, involves evenly distributing the weight onto both legs. The feet are firmly grounded on the floor, drawing energy from the ground, primarily influencing the lower three chakras (root, sacral, and solar plexus chakra; see p. 19).

Muscularly, it primarily targets the shoulders, thighs, and core muscles. The pose opens the hips and enhances knee and hip joint flexibility. Holding *Warrior II* for a more extended period strengthens and stretches the major muscle groups of the legs and chest.

Virabhadrasana II with a strap

Pelvic alignment/alignment of the knee

1.   Create a wide loop in the strap. Step into the strap and assume a wide-leg stance.

2.   Place the right foot on the strap and wrap the other side of the strap around the left shin.

3.   Bend the left leg, ensuring the strap is taut.

4.   Hold the left leg at a right angle and press the outer edge of the right foot into the mat.

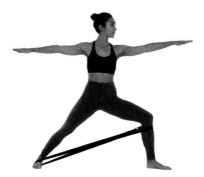

5.   Extend the arms at shoulder height to the sides and look forward over the left arm.

6.   Lift the pelvis and lengthen the spine.

Stay in this pose for up to a minute, deepening your breath into the chest. Come out of the pose and switch sides.

The strap stabilizes the front knee and assists in activating the back leg to achieve balance in the pose. The pelvis remains in its correct alignment, while the erection of the spine may need adjustment.

Virabhadrasana II with a block against the wall

Stabilization of the knee joint

1. Come into Warrior II approximately 25 centimeters away from a wall, with your gaze directed toward the wall.

2. Wedge a block horizontally between the front knee and the wall.

3. Actively press the front leg into the block while allowing the tailbone to relax toward the mat.

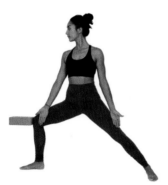

Hold this pose for several deep breaths in Warrior II. Switch sides.

The block prevents overextension of the knee joint beyond a 90-degree angle, activating the supporting back leg and evenly distributing weight on both legs.

Uttitha Trikonasana—Triangle Pose

Utthita = extended, *Tri* = three, Kona = angle

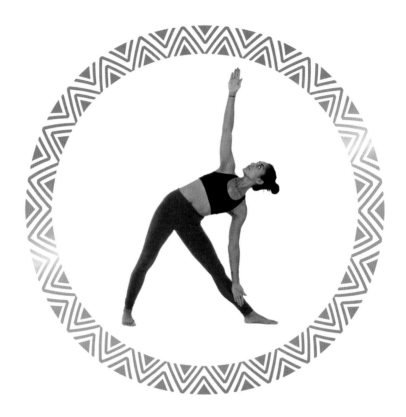

The *Extended Triangle Pose* is among the most intense standing poses, activating and stretching nearly all muscle chains in the body. *Uttitha Trikonasana* enhances spinal flexibility, opens the chest, and strengthens the legs, core, ligaments, and ankles.

It has the potential to alleviate back pain. The firm stance and elongation of the torso over the pelvis specifically targets the root chakra. The expansive posture of the chest guides breath into the heart space, stimulating the *Heart Chakra* (p. 19).

Uttitha Trikonasana with a block

Alignment of the shoulders

1. Place a block upright at the front of the mat.

2. Get into *Uttitha Trikonasana*, bringing the front hand to the block outside the front foot.

3. Extend the upper arm in a vertical line from the block, ensuring precise shoulder alignment.

4. Transfer more weight from the lower hand to the back supporting leg.

5. Open the chest wider.

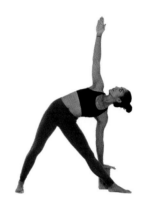

Alternatively, the block can be placed inside the front foot.

Hold this pose for several deep breaths. Exit the pose and switch sides.

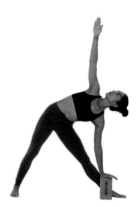

This variation is beneficial for beginners focusing on their alignment. The block supports the lower arm, relieving the lateral core muscles and facilitating proper shoulder alignment.

Utthita Trikonasana with a strap

Activation of the back thigh/chest opening

1. Create a small loop in the strap. Step into the strap with the right foot.

2. Take a big step forward with the left foot, toes pointing straight ahead. The back foot aligns parallel to the end of the mat.

3. Grab the end of the strap with the right hand and extend the arm in line with the shoulder toward the ceiling.

4. Actively push into the outer edge of the back foot, keeping the strap taut above you.

5. Inhale and open up from the back thigh, through the hip, and into the chest.

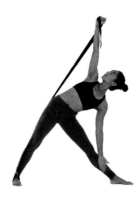

Hold this pose for several deep breaths. Switch sides.

This variation enhances activity in the back leg, the core, and the upper shoulder. It intensifies the opening of the side of the body into the chest and the stretch of the inner side of the front leg.

Parivrtta Trikonasana—Revolved Triangle

Parivrtta = revolved, *Trikona* = three angle, triangle

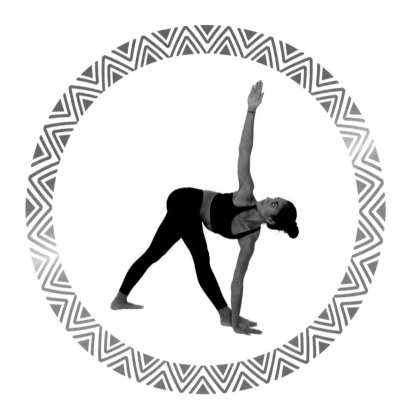

The twisted variation of the *Triangle Pose* is a challenging standing pose that demands both flexibility in the back and a high level of balance. The profound twist of the thoracic spine enhances blood circulation along the spine's nerves. Deep breathing positively influences the blood supply of the abdominal organs during the twist, contributing to overall vitality.

Additionally, as the chest opens, stability and balance are promoted. Avoid this pose in case of back injuries or disc issues.

Parivrtta Trikonasana with a block

Pelvic alignment

1.   Place an upright block at the front of the mat.

2.   Take a step toward the block with the right foot. The toes point straight toward the block. Rotate the left foot 45 degrees outward. The hips face forward. Feet are hip width apart and firmly grounded.

3.   Bring the right hand to the hip. Lift the left arm and stretch your back. Inhale.

4.   Place the left hand on the block. Exhale.

5.   Roll the right shoulder over the left. Inhale. Turn your gaze over the right shoulder.

6.   Extend the right arm. The shoulders are stacked.

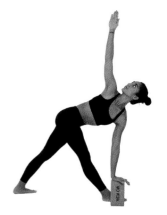

The block can also be placed inside or in front of the front foot as an easier variation.

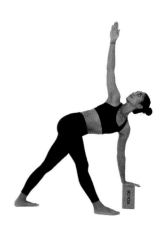

The block helps find balance in the pose, bringing the pelvis into the correct alignment. The extension of the lower arm allows for a wider chest opening.

Parshvakonasana—Extended Side Angle Pose

Utthita = extended, *Parshva* = side, *Kona* = angle

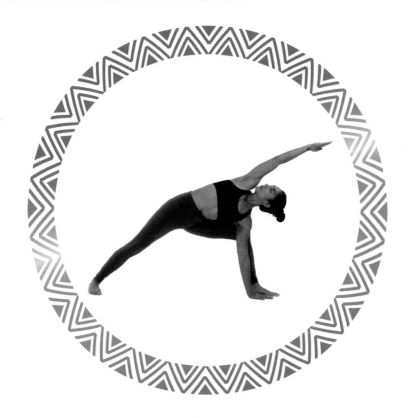

Parsvakonasana is one of the standard poses in Hatha Yoga and, as the name suggests, extends the entire side of the body. The stretch of the body from toes to fingertips opens up the respiratory spaces and provides relief from lower back pain. Thigh muscles and the core are strengthened.

Utthita Parshvakonasana with a block

Knee alignment

1.   Place an upright block at the front of the mat.

2.   Take a big step back with the right leg into a wide stance.

3.   Turn the front foot parallel to the side of the mat. The back foot is parallel to the end of the mat.

4.   Extend the arms at shoulder height to the sides and bend the front leg (see *Virabhadrasana II*, p. 69). The leg forms a 90-degree angle, and the knee should be directly above the ankle.

5.   Lean over the left leg and place the left hand on the block outside the front foot.

6.   Lift the right arm overhead. Stretch the arm as far as possible, maintaining sufficient distance between the shoulder and ear.

7.   The left shoulder should be in a vertical line above the block.

8.   Rotate the back thigh outward and press the outer edge of the back foot firmly into the mat.

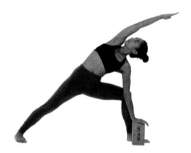

Deeply stretch the entire side of your body and stay in this pose for several deep breaths. Switch sides.

The block serves as an extension of the lower arm and alleviates strain from the front leg. Block support allows for more focus on the lateral stretch of the flank. Be especially mindful not to collapse into the side of the bent leg. The elevation of the block makes it easier to engage the back foot and root deeper into the pose.

Utthita Parshvakonasana with a strap

Side-body stretch

1. Place a strap around the right foot. Hold the end of the strap with the right hand.

2. Take a large step forward with the left leg. Bend the knee at a right angle.

3. Place the left forearm on the thigh and extend the right arm with the strap overhead.

4. Keep the strap taut and actively slide the back foot into the loop.

5. Rotate the back thigh slightly more outward.

6. Stretch the entire right flank, take a deep breath, and try to open the chest further toward the strap.

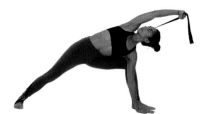 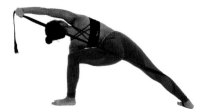

Hold this pose for several deep breaths. The weight is evenly distributed on both legs. Release the strap and come out of the pose. Switch to the other side.

The strap helps keep the back leg actively in external rotation of the thigh, which is crucial for stabilizing the knee joint. Furthermore, holding the strap deepens the stretch along the entire side of the body and opens the chest.

Ardha Chandrasana—Half Moon Pose

Ardha = half, *Chandra* = moon

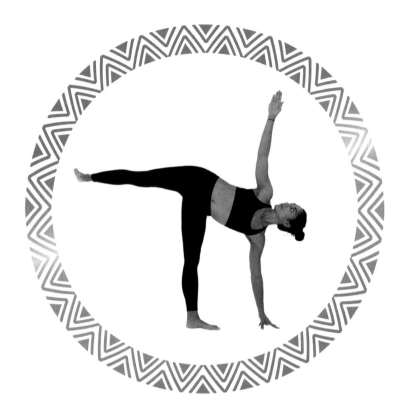

Ardha Chandrasana is a standing balance exercise focusing on training balance and engaging the deep core muscles along the spine. This pose involves stretching the hip, which can be beneficial for alleviating lower back pain and sciatic discomfort. Moreover, the practice strengthens the ankle of the supporting leg, enhancing blood circulation in the foot.

This complex pose engages various muscles in the leg, core, and upper body, contributing to the stability of the root chakra. Additionally, the opening of the hips and shoulders positively influences the heart chakra.

Ardha Chandrasana with a block

Arm alignment

1. Place an upright block at the front of the mat.

2. Take a large step back with the left leg. Move into Warrior II (p. 69).

3. Extend the front arms toward the block. Place the hand on the block. Shift your weight onto the block and lift the back leg.

4. Move the block further forward so the shoulders are aligned.

5. The front foot faces the block. Extend the back leg further and flex the foot in the air. Once you find stability in the pose, open the chest further and look up at the upper arm.

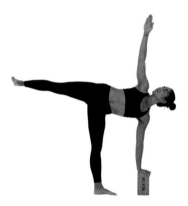

Hold this pose for several deep breaths. Take a big step back into *Warrior II*. Switch sides.

The block serves as an extension of the lower arm and helps with initial balance issues, finding the correct alignment in the pose. If there's stiffness in the lower back, the block aids in opening the hip.

Prasarita Padottanasana—Wide-Leg Forward Bend

Prasarita = outstretched, *Pada* = foot

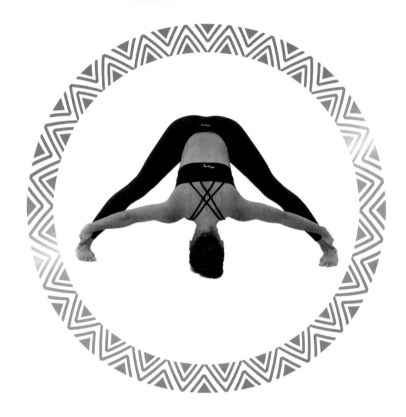

Prasarita Padottanasana has a calming effect on the mind, as the wide stance provides a sense of stability even when bending forward. The hip opening facilitates stretching the lower back into the Forward Bend. This allows the head to relax downward, further loosening the cervical spine.

The backs of the legs are stretched, alleviating lower back pain. Knees and hip joints are strengthened. The root and sacral chakras are opened. Lowering the crown chakra also activates the crown chakra.

Prasarita Padottanasana with a strap

Leg activation/hamstring stretch

1. Create a large loop in the strap. Open your feet wide and tighten the strap around the outer edges of your feet.

2. Keep the strap taut and go deep into the Forward Bend.

3. Try to extend the legs against the strap. Thighs are active.

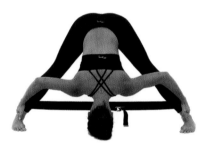

Stay in this pose for several deep breaths (not longer than a minute). Bring your hands to your hips and, with a long back, return to an upright position, lifting the head last.

The strap makes it easier to press the outer edges of the feet into the mat. Since the strap is held taut, the thighs and abductors are automatically engaged. This adds compactness to the pelvis, preventing the feet from slipping. The stretch in the back of the thighs is intensified.

Prasarita Padottanasana with two blocks

Deepening the Forward Bend

1.   Place the two flat blocks at the distance of a wide stance.

2.   Stand on the blocks.

3.   Press the feet actively into the blocks. Activate the thighs. Make sure the blocks can't slip.

4.   Bring your hands to the hips and slowly bend forward.

5.   Place the hands on the outside of the ankles and lengthen the crown of the head toward the floor.

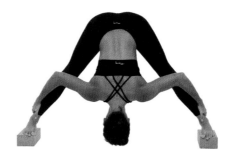

The blocks serve as an extension of the legs, assisting in an intense stretch of the backs of the legs. This variation benefits individuals with a long upper body to go deeper into the Forward Bend. The spine, especially the lower back, can be stretched more effectively.

Prasarita Padottanasana Twist with a block

Chest opening

1. Place a flat block along the long side of the mat.

2. Get into a wide stance with the feet parallel to the short edges of the mat.

3. Bring your hands on your hips and bend forward with a long spine.

4. Place the left hand on the block. Inhale and lift the right arm. The hands are aligned in a vertical line. Open the chest.

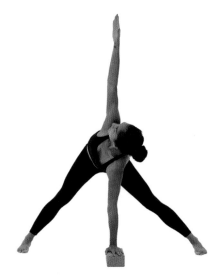

Stay in this pose for several deep breaths. Return to the center and switch sides.

The blocks serve as an extension of the arms, allowing for further chest opening without compromising pelvic alignment. The twist is also felt as a stretch in the hips and the insides of the legs.

Parsvottanasana—Intense Side Stretch

Parsva = side, *Uttana* = stretch

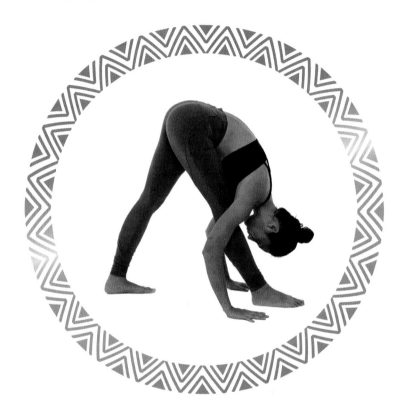

Parsvottanasana, often known as Pyramid Pose, is among the forward-bending standing poses that stretch not only both sides of the torso but also the chest and flanks. It enhances balance.

The posture's alignment is crucial to creating a stable foundation and fully experiencing *Parsvottanasana's* benefits. Blocks can be very helpful for a secure stance.

Parsvottanasana with two blocks

Pelvic alignment

1. Place two upright blocks at the front of the mat.

2. Take a medium-sized step back with the left foot, turning it about 45 degrees outward.

3. Keep both feet firmly on the ground and bring your hands to your hips. Inhale, lengthen the spine and bend forward with a straight back.

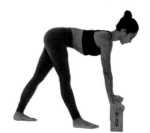

4. Place your hands on the upright blocks, aligning them under your shoulders.

5. Gently draw the right hip back, keeping the pelvis aligned. The front leg is slightly bent, and both thighs are evenly activated.

6. Exhale and bend forward into the stretch.

Hold this pose for a few deep breaths. Come back up with a long spine and switch sides.

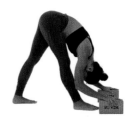

This variation is especially suitable for beginners who struggle with balance. The blocks assist in finding balance for a stable posture. As an extension of the arms, they aid in pelvic alignment and stabilizing the feet on the ground.

Parsvottanasana with a strap

Shoulder opening

1.   Hold a strap in your right hand.

2.   Take a medium-sized step back with the left foot, turning it about 45 degrees outward. Feet are hip width apart.

3.   Raise the right arm overhead, bending it so the long end of the strap is hanging down.

4.   Slightly open the left arm to the side, palm facing forward.

5.   Tilt the left shoulder forward, turning the palm backward.

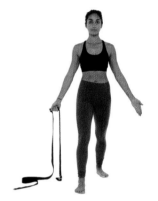

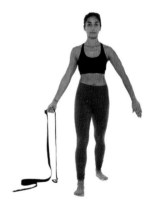

6.   Bend the left arm, reaching behind your back for the lower end of the strap.

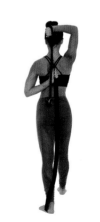

7.   Pull on both ends of the strap, extending your spine as much as possible.

8.   Keep the front leg slightly bent. Inhale, lean forward with a long back.

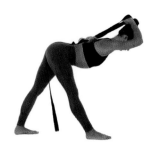

9.   Exhale and sink deeper into the stretch. Maintain tension on the strap. Keep the chest open.

Hold this pose for a few deep breaths. Maintain tension on the strap and slowly rise. Switch sides.

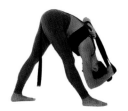

This variation suits advanced practitioners seeking to deepen the flank stretch and chest opening. The strap ensures spinal length and enhances shoulder joint mobility. The upper back is stabilized in this pose.

Virabhadrasana III—Warrior III

Vira = brave, *Bhadra* = gracious

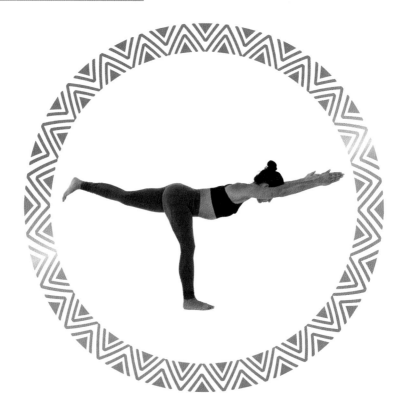

Warrior III symbolizes calm, serenity, and inner balance, as unlike *Virabhadrasana I and II*, it is performed on one leg. The hips are closed to maintain balance. Like in a standing scale, the small stabilizing muscles must keep the spine horizontally aligned. In addition to balance, intrinsic muscles are trained.

The ankle and thighs of the supporting leg are strengthened, which activates the core muscles. The head's position in line with the spine effectively trains the sense of balance in the inner ear.

Virabhadrasana III with two blocks

Pelvic alignment

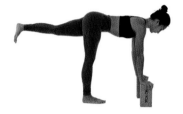

1. Place two blocks upright at the front of the mat.

2. Move into a Half-Forward Bend, hands on the upright blocks. The blocks are directly under the shoulders.

3. Focus on a steady point on the ground, keeping the neck long.

4. Slowly lift the left leg, keeping the hips closed, and the leg actively extended. The foot is flexed, and the toes point straight down.

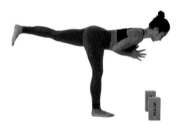

5. Keep the supporting leg active, and draw the chest forward to lengthen the spine. The lower foot is facing straight, with toes to the front.

6. Once you find balance, slowly release your hands from the blocks, bringing them to the heart. Palms together, with the thumb gently pushing the chest back.

Hold this pose for a few deep breaths. Slowly place the left foot down next to the right. Switch sides.

*This variation is particularly suitable for beginners working on their sense of balance. The challenge in **Warrior III** is keeping the hips closed while lifting the leg to avoid overarching. The blocks serve as an extension of the arms, assisting in finding balance and maintaining proper pelvic alignment. This helps to elongate the spine.*

Virabhadrasana III with a strap

Activation of the lifted leg/spinal stretch

1. Secure the strap above your left knee, grasping the end with both hands behind your body.

2. Take a large step forward with your right foot.

3. Extend your reach for the strap over the inside of your left leg, pulling gently to encourage further outward thigh rotation.

4. As you inhale, draw the end of the strap overhead with both hands. Extend your left leg back behind you, transitioning into *Virabhadrasana III.I*.

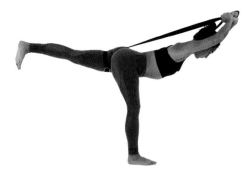

5. Maintain tension in the strap while keeping your upper body parallel to the mat. Reach your arms overhead, allowing your shoulder blades to draw inward and your chest to expand. Actively engage the back heel by pushing it backward while lifting the leg to align with your spine. Ensure that your hips remain squared.

Stay in this pose for a few deep breaths. Keep the strap taut to stretch the spine further. Switch sides.

This modification enhances **Warrior III** *for advanced practitioners. The strap aids in maintaining the lifted back leg by engaging the arms and upper back muscles. It encourages spinal elongation, fosters chest expansion, and reinforces the shoulder girdle.*

Utkatasana—Chair Pose

Utkata = immense, superior

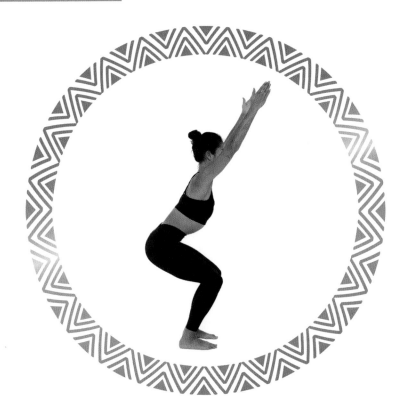

Translated, *Utkatasana* means the powerful or vigorous posture. Fully engaging the thighs is essential in the bent leg position, while spinal extension implies activating the core muscles.

In the full pose, the arms extend forward, facilitating a deeper stretch of the sides of the torso. Activation of major muscles in the body stimulates the cardiovascular system, enhancing blood circulation. Opening up the respiratory spaces stimulates the heart chakra.

Utkatasana with a block

Activation of the thighs/pelvic alignment

1.   Begin by placing a block between the inner thighs.

2.   Bend the knees and extend the arms forward to come into *Utkatasana*. Lengthen the tailbone toward the heels and open the chest. Ensure the knees are bent over the middle of the foot arch, avoiding extension beyond the toes.

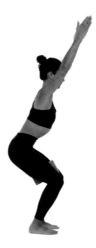

Hold this pose for a few deep breaths. Actively press your inner thighs into the block. Slowly lower the arms and straighten the legs to release the pose.

The goal of the pose is to maintain length in the lower back while opening the chest. Holding the block strengthens the adductors on the inner thighs and assists beginners in lifting the pelvis without arching the lower back..

Utkatasana Twist with a block

Pelvic alignment/mobility of the thoracic spine

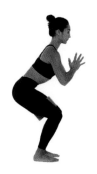

1. Begin by placing a block between the inner thighs.

2. Press the palms together and bring the hands to your heart.

3. Bend the knees and twist the upper body to the right.

4. Lengthen the spine and deepen the bend to bring the left elbow to the outside of the right thigh.

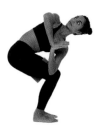

5. Inhale, lengthening the upper back. Push the chest toward your thumbs.

6. Exhale, twisting the chest further to the right. Hold the block firmly between the thighs. Keep the pelvis straight as the torso twists over the thoracic spine.

Hold this pose for a few deep breaths. Slowly rotate the upper body back to the center and straighten up. Switch sides.

The challenge of the twisted chair pose lies in maintaining a straight pelvis while the upper body twists. Holding the block allows for a twist isolated from the lower part of the body, focusing on the thoracic spine.

Open Twist with a block

Chest opening/stretching the outer thigh

1. Begin by placing a block upright at the front of the mat.

2. Rest the left hand on it, aligning the block with the left shoulder.

3. Bend the left knee and extend the right arm upward. The chest opens, and the arms are in a vertical line to each other.

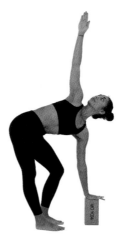

Hold this pose for a few deep breaths. Rotate the upper body without losing the grounding of the right foot. Slowly turn back down and switch to the other side.

The block acts as an extension of the lower arm, facilitating further chest opening without neglecting pelvic alignment. Additionally, the outer thigh experiences an intense stretch.

Natarajasana—Dancer Pose

Nata = dancer, *Raja* = king

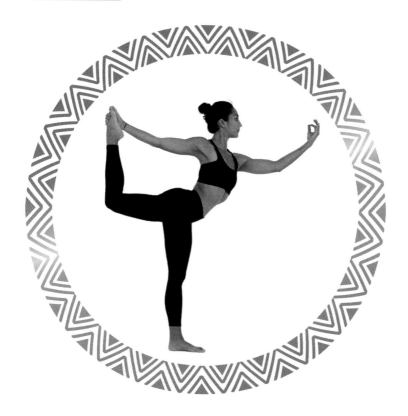

Natajarasana is dedicated to the Hindu god Shiva, known in Indian mythology as an extraordinary dancer. This advanced yoga pose combines a Backbend with a balancing posture, demanding significant physical strength and mental patience. When executed correctly, it enhances balance, stretches the front body, and opens the groin, abdomen, and heart space. It stimulates the root, sacral, and particularly the heart chakra.

Overall, the *Dancer Pose* harmonizes the system, providing physical and mental stability. Avoiding this pose in cases of acute back pain or knee issues is advisable.

Natajarasana with a strap

Chest opening/strengthening thighs and shoulder girdle

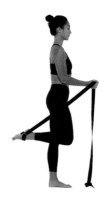

1.   Begin by creating a small loop in the strap and placing it around your right foot.

2.   Grip the long end of the strap with your right hand.

3.   Bend your right leg, drawing the heel toward your right buttock.

4.   Drape the strap over your left shoulder and extend your right hand over your head, securing the strap with both hands.

5.   Activate your supporting leg and gently lean your upper body forward, using the strap to guide the lifted leg higher.

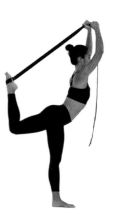

Hold this pose for a few deep breaths, then gradually release your hands from the strap, first the right, then the left, and switch sides.

This variation is tailored for advanced practitioners aiming to deepen the Backbend. Adjusting the grip on the strap allows for a higher leg lift, intensifying the front body's opening and fortifying the shoulder girdle. By actively pressing the foot into the loop, you engage the thigh muscles for added support.

Ushtrasana—Camel Pose

Ushtra = camel

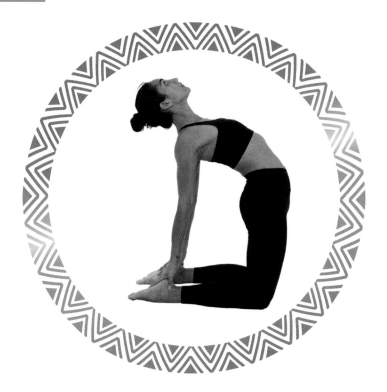

Camel Pose is a demanding Backbend carried out from a kneeling position, necessitating significant involvement of the back, spine, and especially the core muscles.

This posture elongates the front of the body, stretching the chest and shoulders while activating the respiratory muscles to expand the breathing passages. Lung capacity is boosted, and the internal organs receive a beneficial stimulus.

From an energetic standpoint, this pose predominantly influences the heart and throat chakras. Emotionally, *Ushtrasana* fosters self-confidence by baring the vulnerable areas of the heart and abdomen.

It's essential to approach *Ushtrasana* with care and practice it only when no injuries or acute back issues are present. With a healthy spine and proper execution, *Ushtrasana* can be a preventive measure against future back problems by strengthening the internal supporting muscles.

Ushtrasana with two blocks

Support of the back

1. Start by placing two upright blocks shoulder width apart in the center of your mat.

2. Come into a kneeling position with your back facing the blocks and your toes planted firmly on the mat.

3. Bring your hands to your lower back and gradually lean your upper back backward, ensuring your pelvis stays aligned over your knees and your abdominal muscles remain engaged.

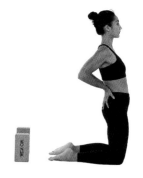

4. Activate your gluteal muscles and slowly release your hands from your back.

5. Place your hands on the blocks, positioning them directly under your shoulders.

6. Roll your shoulder blades inward and gently allow your head to drop back.

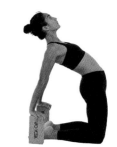

7. As you inhale, lift your chest higher, and as you exhale, gently push your pelvis forward.

Remain in this pose for a few deep breaths. Slowly bring your hands back to your lower back, lift your head, and use your engaged abdominal muscles to get the rest of your upper body up. Transition into *Child's Pose* (p.150) for balance.

The blocks act as an extension of the arms, enabling advanced practitioners to deepen their Backbend before progressing to the complete variation where the hands touch the heels. For beginners, especially those with shortened quadriceps, the blocks offer excellent support to approach the full expression of the pose.

Navasana—Boat Pose

Nava = boat

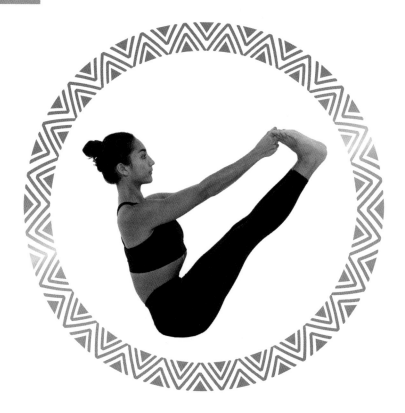

Navasana is a balancing pose executed in a seated position, primarily challenging the core muscles while maintaining balance on the sit bones. The lower abdomen plays a crucial role in preserving the length of the lower back, while the hip flexors actively engage to support the leg weight.

Energetically, the Boat Pose symbolizes stability in the root chakra and emphasizes the power of the core within the solar plexus chakra. Mentally, practicing *Navasana* enhances concentration and fosters perseverance. For individuals dealing with back issues or those with weaker core muscles, it is advisable to consider performing a Half Boat Pose with bent legs.

Navasana with a block

Activation of pelvic floor muscles/hip flexors

1. Begin in a seated position with both feet grounded on the floor, ensuring the spine is aligned directly above the pelvis.

2. Place a block between your thighs.

3. Grasp the outer sides of the thighs with your hands and lean back while maintaining an elongated spine.

4. Gradually lift your feet off the mat, maintaining a secure grip on the block between your thighs.

5. Achieve balance on the sit bones, extending your arms forward with a focused gaze toward the big toes while flexing your feet.

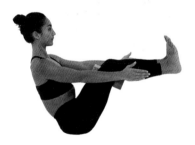

Stay in this pose for a few deep breaths, then slowly lower your feet back to the mat.

The block helps to engage the inner thighs, hip flexors, and the deep pelvic floor muscles essential for balance and leg support.

Navasana with a strap

Relief of the lower back

1.   Begin by sitting upright with your feet on the mat in front of you.

2.   Place a wide strap around your upper back and the soles of your feet, ensuring the buckle is conveniently accessible on the side.

3.   Engage your core muscles and lift your legs, adjusting the strap width if necessary.

4.   Gradually push the soles of your feet into the strap to straighten your legs.

5.   Find balance on your sit bones, maintaining an upright spine as you lean back into the strap.

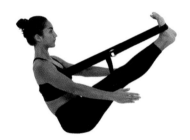

Remain in this pose for as long as it feels comfortable.

The strap facilitates achieving the full expression of the pose without the weight of the legs straining your abdomen and lower back, offering relief to the lower back.

Setu Bandhasana—Bridge Pose

Setu = bridge / *Bandha* = bond, arrest

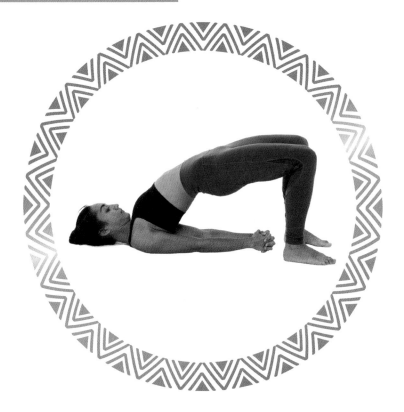

The *Bridge Pose*, also called the *Half-Wheel*, seamlessly blends an inverted position with a Backbend. Energetically, it brings both refreshing and calming effects, offering a milder alternative to *Urdhva Dhanurasana*—the Wheel (p. 107).

Primarily targeting the heart and throat chakras, the Bridge Pose fortifies the solar plexus and root chakras. Engaged muscles encompass the core, back, thighs, and glutes.

The elevation of the pelvis strengthens the back and elongates the front of the body. The chosen arm variation may influence the expansion of the shoulders and chest.

Setu Bandhasana with a block under the sacrum

Supporting the Bridge Pose

1.   Prepare a block and lie on your back. Position your feet a hand's length in front of your buttocks.

2.   Lift the pelvis into *Setu Bandhasana* and slide the block under the sacrum. Adjust the block's position based on the desired intensity, either flat or upright.

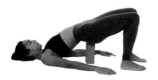 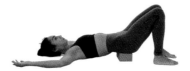

3.   Rest your pelvis on the block.

Stay in this pose for a few deep breaths. To deepen the Backbend, you can extend your arms overhead.

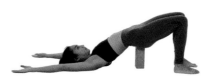

Press both feet actively into the mat, lifting your hips. Move the block aside and slowly roll your back down on the mat. For lower back relief, draw your knees toward your chest.

Supported Bridge Pose offers a beautiful transition from muscular passivity to feeling the energetic impact of the pose. It effortlessly opens up the respiratory spaces, and the body naturally takes the shape of the Backbend.

For a more stable base, you can place two blocks flat under the pelvis as an alternative.

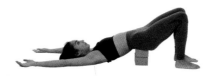

Setu Bandhasana with a strap

Chest opening

1.   Sit up straight with your feet positioned a hand's length in front of your buttocks.

2.   Secure a strap around your ankles, just above them.

3.   Lie on your back.

4.   Elevate your hips to enter Bridge Pose.

5.   Maintain tension in both ends of the strap to enhance the Backbend.

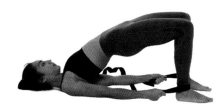

Stay in this pose for a few deep breaths, inhaling deeply into your chest. Roll your spine back down to the mat, releasing the strap. Allow your knees to gently come together at the center and feel the effects of the pose.

The strap amplifies the chest opening in the Backbend and engages the thigh muscles for added strength.

Urdhva Dhanurasana—Wheel Pose

Urdhva = upward, *Dhanur* = arch

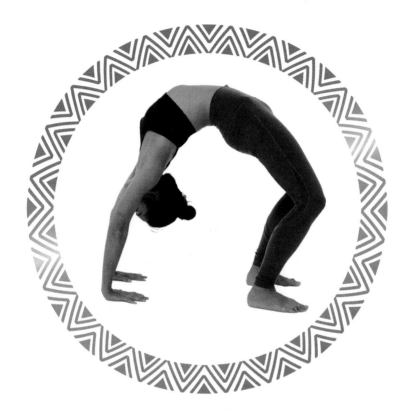

Urdhva Dhanurasana is one of the most challenging Backbends, requiring physical strength, flexibility, courage, and willpower. If your shoulders and back are strong enough to lift the pelvis, the spine arches like a bow, stretching the entire front body and creating more space for the organs. It strengthens and keeps the spine supple.

The inversion of the head addresses the solar plexus, heart chakra, and third eye chakra.

Inverting Backbends like *Urdhva Dhanurasana* enhance self-confidence and invigorate the nervous system. Avoid practicing it before bedtime or with migraines, headaches, or high/low blood pressure.

If you have acute back issues or injuries, skip this pose. Instead, practice the Bridge Pose.

Urdhva Dhanurasana with two blocks against the wall

Relief of the shoulders/wrists

1. Position two blocks diagonally and shoulder width apart against a wall, ensuring the blocks and the mat underneath are non-slip.

2. Lie on your back with your head facing the wall, aligning your shoulders in front of the blocks.

3. Place your feet parallel to each other, maintaining a hand's length distance from the buttocks, with a fist-width gap between the knees.

4. Rest your hands on the blocks, fingers turned toward your body.

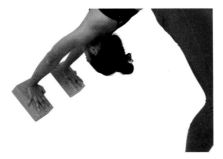

5. Press the blocks firmly into the wall and lift the pelvis, moving into a complete Wheel Pose.

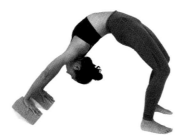

The diagonal hand positioning provides a soothing effect on the wrists, particularly beneficial for those with shortened muscles in the front body, promoting correct hand alignment. The counterpressure against the wall also lends support to the shoulders while intensifying the stretch across the chest and abdominal muscles.

Urdhva Dhanurasana with a strap

Pelvic alignment

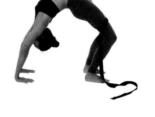

1.   Begin by lying on your back with your feet set hip width apart.

2.   Loop the strap just above the knees, securing it around your thighs.

3.   Position your hands close to your ears on the mat, with fingertips pointing toward your feet.

4.   Simultaneously press into your hands and feet, lifting the pelvis while resting the crown of the head on the mat.

5.   Roll back your shoulder blades and press the outer thighs into the strap.

6.   Elevate the pelvis higher and gradually release the head from the mat to move into *Urdhva Dhanurasana*, ensuring the strap remains taut.

Hold the pose for a few deep breaths. Slowly bend your arms, place the crown of the head on the ground, lower the chin to the chest, and roll down vertebra by vertebra. Allow the knees to sink together in the middle to alleviate the lower back, taking a moment to feel the effect of the posture.

Entering the wheel requires considerable effort, simultaneously engaging the shoulders, arms, back, and legs. This may occasionally compromise proper alignment.

The strap prevents the knees from tipping to the sides, ensuring the pelvis maintains alignment and facilitating maximum hip flexor and thigh stretching.

The engagement of the thigh and hip surrounding muscles, coupled with the tension on the strap, safeguards the lower back during the deep Backbend.

Salamba Sarvangasana—Shoulder Stand

Salamba = supported, *sarva* = all, *anga* = limb, part

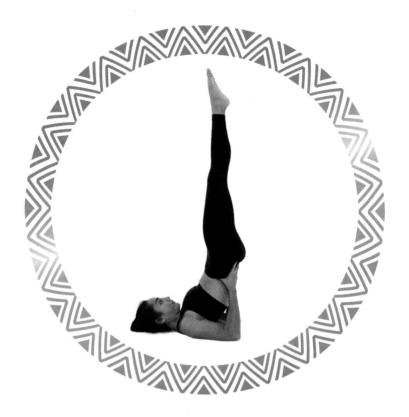

The Supported Shoulder Stand is a standard inversion pose in advanced yoga and is usually practiced toward the end of the session due to its energetic effects. It stimulates digestion and lymphatic flow, preparing the body for post-yoga recovery.

Energetically, *Salamba Sarvangasana* mainly activates the throat chakra. It should never be practiced with injuries in the cervical spine or stiffness in the neck. Particularly in the early stages, incorporating props into the pose can prevent injuries or incorrect execution.

Salamba Sarvangasana with a blanket

Shoulder alignment/relief of the cervical spine

1. Carefully fold a blanket into a square. The edges should be even and straight.

2. Lie on your back. Place the head just at the edge of the blanket and align the shoulder blades with the upper edge of the blanket. Feet are planted in front of the hips, arms close to the body with palms facing up.

3. Pull the bent legs toward the body. Activate the abdominal muscles, rolling the pubic bone inward.

4. With some momentum—but using primarily lower abdominal strength—lift the pelvis and bring your hands to the lower back. Bring the knees toward the head.

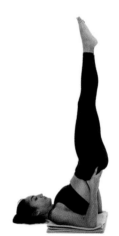

5. Slide your hands toward the middle of the back, thumbs pointing forward, and fingers toward the spine.

6. Bring the shoulders and torso closer together until the chest touches the chin.

7. Slowly begin to straighten the legs. The spine is aligned directly above the pelvis, the tailbone drawing inward, and the elbows staying close together.

Hold this pose for several deep breaths. Bend the legs, bring the thighs to the belly, slowly lower the buttocks, release the hands, and roll the back down onto the mat, one vertebra at a time.

The blanket provides a platform for the shoulders, supporting the body's weight and maintaining the correct posture. It protects the protruding spinous process of the cervical and thoracic spine and prevents overextension of the cervical spine.

Halasana—Plow

Hala = plow

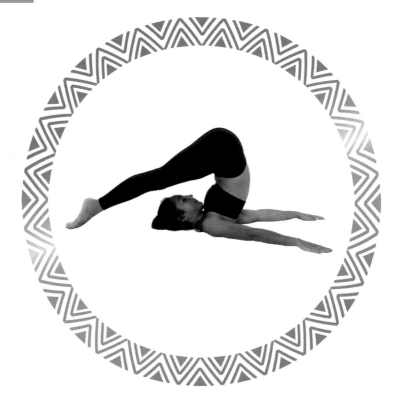

The Plow is an ancient tool used for farming, symbolizing work, patience, and preparing the ground for transformation and growth.

Like the Shoulder Stand, the Plow has a highly energetic effect. Since the inversion doesn't require active shoulder or abdominal muscle strength, it harmonizes and balances the system. The spine becomes more flexible, and the sciatic nerve is stretched.

This can relieve lower back discomfort, as sciatic pain often radiates to the lower back. *Halasana* has a stimulating and simultaneously calming effect on the energy system, particularly on the throat chakra. It should not be practiced in cases of acute neck issues, injuries to the cervical spine, or shoulder stiffness.

Halasana with a blanket and a block

Shoulder alignment/relief of the cervical spine

1. Fold a blanket carefully into a square at the beginning of your mat. The edges of the blanket should be even and straight.

2. Place a block in the center at the end of the mat.

3. Lie down on your back. The head is positioned at the edge of the blanket. The shoulder blades align with the blanket's top edge, and the crown of the head is aligned with the block. Feet are planted on the floor. Arms lie close to the body with palms facing up.

4. Draw the bent legs toward your body. Activate the abdominal muscles and roll the pubic bone backward.

5. With momentum and using strength primarily from the lower abdomen, bring your legs over your head, placing the toes on the block.

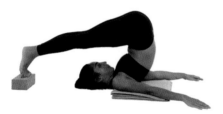

Stay in this pose for a few deep breaths. Bend the legs, bringing the thighs toward the chest. Slowly lower the buttocks, release the hands, and roll the spine down, vertebra by vertebra, onto the mat.

The support of the blanket and block aids individuals with limited mobility in achieving the pose. Placing the shoulders on the blanket relieves pressure on the lumbar spine. Elevating the feet on the block reduces the legs' weight against gravity.

5
SUPPORTED
Stretches

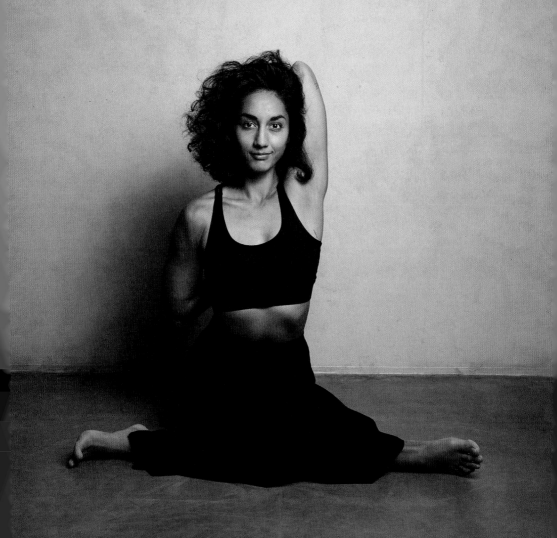

Dandasana—Staff Pose

Danda = staff

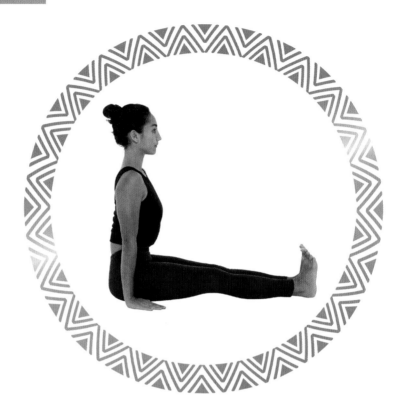

Dandasana is considered the standard seated pose and serves as the starting position for yoga poses like *Paschimottanasana*, the seated Forward Bend (p. 137), which requires length in the lower back. Emphasizing pelvic alignment, *Dandasana* establishes the groundwork for lengthening the lower back and the entire spine. Beyond engaging the muscles in the back and abdomen, it activates the deep muscles in the pelvic floor.

The straight posture and inner alignment counteract a slouched posture, often a cause for back pain. The spine elongates, and the two posterior sides are actively stretched, which can help alleviate sciatic discomfort. *Dandasana* is excellent for preparing the mind for mat practice, requiring mental focus, and assisting with inner restlessness. Energetically, it primarily influences the root chakra. However, the activation of abdominal muscles also addresses the solar plexus chakra. The sought alignment of the spine further establishes a connection to the crown chakra.

Dandasana with a blanket and two blocks

Pelvic alignment/spinal stretch

1. Sit up straight on a neatly folded blanket. Position two flat blocks on either side of the pelvis.

2. Place your hands flat on the blocks, ensuring your wrists are aligned under the shoulders.

3. Stretch your legs out lengthwise. Flex your feet and press your heels into the mat.

4. Actively push your hands into the blocks, almost lifting your buttocks off the blanket. Gently draw your shoulders back, keeping your neck relaxed.

5. Use the strength of your lower abdominal muscles to straighten and further lengthen your spine.

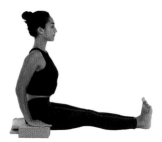

Remain in this pose for a few deep breaths.

The folded blanket aids in pelvic alignment and provides relief to the Achilles tendons. The blocks assist in extending the torso, which can be particularly beneficial for individuals with shorter arms.

Dandasana with a block

Pelvic alignment/activation of the pelvic floor muscles

1.   Sit upright on a block laid flat.

2.   Position your fingertips just behind the shoulders next to the block. Draw the shoulder blades together and keep the spine upright.

3.   Extend your legs lengthwise. Flex your feet and actively press the heels into the ground.

4.   Lift the pelvis and engage the pelvic floor muscles, lifting the lower back out of the pelvis like a lift.

5.   Draw the crown of the head toward the ceiling. Over time, you can lift the fingertips a few centimeters from the ground. Aim to maintain the lower back in an upright position.

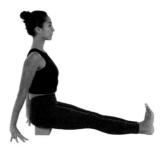

Remain in this pose for a few deep breaths.

This variation is particularly beneficial for beginners working on abdominal muscle strength or those with shortened hamstrings. Sitting elevated on the block aids in pelvic alignment and promotes a straight spine.

Dandasana with a strap

Spinal stretch/stretching the back of the legs/shoulder opening

1.   Move into an upright seated position.

2.   Bring your feet up and loop a strap around the soles of your feet, gripping the long ends with both hands.

3.   Ensure both sit bones are evenly grounded on the mat. Slowly slide the soles of your feet into the strap while straightening your legs.

4.   Keep the thigh muscles engaged and the pelvis upright. Roll the shoulder blades back to straighten the spine further. Hold this pose for a few deep breaths, focusing on breathing deeply into the muscle heads.

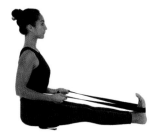

Stay in this pose for several deep breaths.

The support of the strap is especially beneficial for individuals with shortened hamstrings. Holding the strap enhances the activity of the back extensors and promotes an upright position in the upper body.

Dandasana with a strap

Pelvic alignment/activation of the legs/stretching the back of the legs

1.   Move into an upright seated position. Place a widely looped strap around the pelvis and the soles of the feet. Your lower back is well anchored in the pelvis, and the legs are slightly bent but active. The feet are apart and pointing outward.

2.   Place the hands on the floor and slowly begin to straighten the legs.

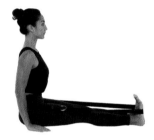

Stay in this pose for a few deep breaths.

This variation is especially suitable for beginners struggling with pelvic alignment. The strap offers support in achieving the hamstring stretch, creating a framework that stabilizes the pelvis. This, in turn, reduces the workload on the pelvic muscles. Breath can flow more deeply into the abdominal area, promoting the massage of organs and stimulating digestion.

Dandasana with a block

Stretching the back of the legs

1. Place a block flat at the end of the mat.

2. Come into an upright seat, extend the legs, and place the heels on the block.

3. Keep your feet slightly open and flexed, and actively press the heels into the block.

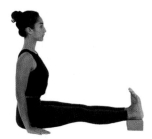

Stay in this pose for a few deep breaths.

Pressing the heels into the blocks activates the thighs and intensifies the stretch in the hamstrings. The pelvis can be better aligned.

Baddha Konasana—Seated Angle Pose

Baddha = bound, *Kona* = angle

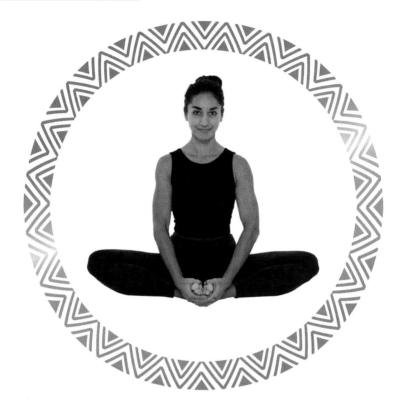

Baddha Konasana, often called the Butterfly Pose, is a hip-opening seated asana stretching the groins and hip flexors.

The support of the abdominal muscles in pelvic alignment promotes blood circulation in the abdominal organs, offering relief during menstruation. The hip opening facilitates the upright positioning of the lower back.

Baddha Konasana is good preparation for seated Forward Bends like *Paschimottanasana* (p. 137) or *Upavistha Konasana* (p. 127). Energetically, the hip opening primarily influences the root and sacral chakras associated with sexuality and reproduction.

Baddha Konasana with a block

Pelvic alignment/hip opening

1. Sit on a flat block or a folded blanket or cushion.

2. Bring the soles of your feet together and let the knees drop to the sides.

3. Grip both feet with your hands. Roll the inner edges of the feet outward, intensifying the stretch in the inner thighs. The outer edges of the feet continue to touch..

4. Roll the shoulders away from the ears and further straighten the spine.

5. Inhale and lengthen the spine. Exhale, allowing the knees to descend closer to the mat. Stay in this pose for several deep breaths.

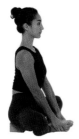 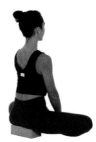

This variation is especially suitable for beginners working on hip opening. If, for instance, the hip muscles are tight, causing the knees to be above the pelvis, the elevation from the block aids pelvic alignment and intensifies the groin stretch.

Baddha Konasana with two blocks

Pelvic alignment/stretching the inside of the legs

1. Place two flat blocks shoulder width apart at the end of the mat, with their long sides aligned vertically to the mat's long sides.

2. Come into *Baddha Konasana* with your back facing the blocks.

3. Place your hands behind you on the blocks.

4. Push both hands into the blocks, lifting the buttocks off the floor. Move the pelvis slightly forward until the buttocks almost touch the heels.

5. Lower the buttocks back down.

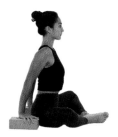

Stay in this pose for several deep breaths.

The blocks allow you to bring the pelvis closer to the heels, intensifying the stretch on both inner sides and opening the groins in the final position.

Baddha Konasana with a blanket and a strap

Pelvic alignment/centering of the hips

1. Come into *Baddha Konasana* (p 122). Place a strap around the outer edges of your feet and the pelvis. Ensure the buckle is in front and easily accessible.

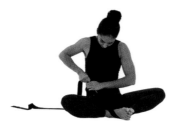

2. Adjust your feet with both hands. Allow the knees to drop to the sides and into the strap.

3. Continue lifting the pelvis and straightening your spine.

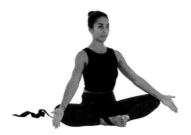

Stay in this pose for several deep breaths.

The strap compacts the pelvis, allowing deeper hip opening and spine elongation. Holding the knees against the resistance of the strap deepens the stretch in the groins and inner thighs.

Baddha Konasana with a block

Hip opening/groin stretch

1.   Come into *Baddha Konasana.*

2.   Place a block vertically between the soles of your feet.

3.   Grip your feet from the outside, press the soles into the block, and roll the inner thighs outward.

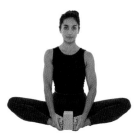

Stay in this pose for several deep breaths.

The thigh bone is actively pressed into the hip socket by pushing the feet into the block. The thighs can rotate outward, intensifying the stretch in the groins.

Upavistha Konasana—Wide Straddle

Upavishta = seated, *Kona* = angle

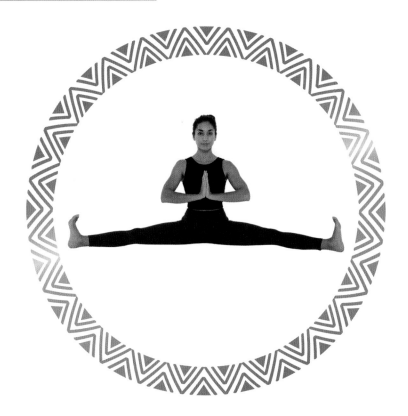

Upavistha Konasana, also referred to as the *Wide-Angle Seated Forward Bend*, is a staple among seated hip-opening poses. The act of spreading the legs provides relief from sciatic discomfort and tension in the abdomen. This pose effectively stretches the inner thighs and groin area.

On an energetic level, practicing this seated angle stimulates the root and sacral chakras, particularly emphasizing the sacral region. This stimulation occurs as the pose opens the pelvic area and encourages deep belly breathing, thus activating the reproductive organs.

Upavistha Konasana with a blanket

Pelvic alignment

1. Sit on the front edge of a carefully folded blanket.

2. Spread your legs into a wide-angle stretch. Feet are flexed, toes pointing upwards.

3. Place your fingertips on the inside of your thighs. Stay evenly grounded on both sit bones while straightening the pelvis and lower back.

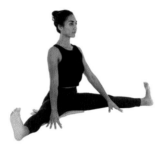

Stay in this pose for several deep breaths.

Sitting elevated on the blanket supports pelvic alignment, improving lower back extension. The alignment of the toes serves as a guide to ensure the pelvis is upright—ideally, the toes should point directly upward.

Upavistha Konasana with two straps

Pelvic alignment/core stabilization

1. Start by coming into a wide-angle stretch.

2. Place a strap around each foot.

3. Bend your knees and hold the ends of the straps with both hands. Roll your shoulder blades back and lift over the pelvis.

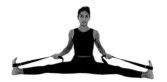

4. Begin sliding your feet into the straps and slowly straighten your legs.

5. Gradually pull on the ends of the straps to lift the lower back further and elongate the spine.

Alternatively, you can hold the straps crossed.

Stay in this pose for several deep breaths. Keep the straps taut and the pelvis aligned.

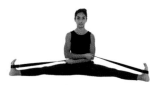

This variation is well-suited for advanced practitioners seeking to deepen the stretch's intensity. pulling on the straps engages the inner thighs and quadriceps, aligning the torso over the pelvic base.

Upavistha Konasana with two blocks

Stretching the inside of the legs/activation of the quadriceps

1. Place two blocks flat at the short ends of the mat.

2. Spread your legs into a wide-angle stretch. Position your hands behind your hips and rest your heels on the blocks, ensuring your feet remain flexed.

3. Press your palms firmly into the ground, engaging your core to lift the torso. Pull up on the kneecaps and rotate the thighs outward, allowing the pelvis to rise.

4. Lift the chest and roll the shoulder blades back as you inhale, elongating the spine.

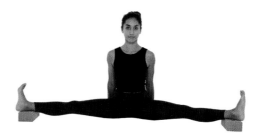

Hold this pose for several deep breaths in *Upavistha Konasana*.

This variation of the stretch is ideal for experienced practitioners seeking to deepen the pose and enhance the stretch in their legs. Elevating the heels activates and strengthens the quadriceps, adding an extra layer of intensity to the posture.

Swastikasana—Auspicious Pose

Swastika = well-being

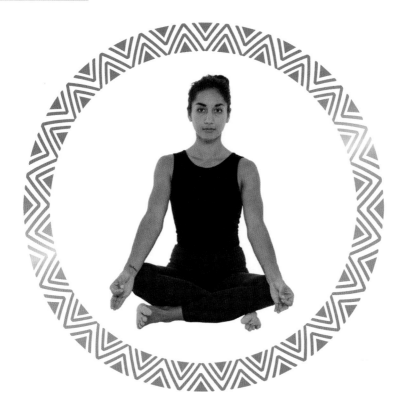

Swastikasana is considered one of the foundational poses in Hatha Yoga, serving as an active seated posture for meditation. Mentally, it brings a clarifying effect to the mind.

Physically, it enhances hip and groin flexibility while promoting overall blood circulation in the legs, relieving discomfort or fatigue. This seated posture with crossed legs primarily engages the root and sacral chakras.

In a meditative state, consciously aligning the spine activates all energy centers. However, individuals experiencing chronic or acute knee issues should opt for an alternative meditation pose, such as the Hero Pose (p.147).

Swastikasana with two blocks and a blanket

Pelvic alignment/lower back straightening/chest and shoulder opening

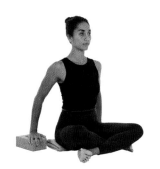

1.   Begin by sitting on a carefully folded blanket with your legs extended and slightly apart.

2.   Use your hands to roll the fronts of your thighs in, feeling the sit bones widen, allowing you to lift through their center.

3.   Bend your right leg and left, crossing the middle of the shins with the feet under the knees.

4.   Place two blocks on either side of the blanket.

5.   Rest your hands on the blocks, actively pressing your fingertips into them, and lifting the buttocks slightly. Relax the groin, allowing the pelvis to sink naturally. Lower the sit bones onto the blanket.

6.   Roll the shoulders away from the ears, placing the backs of your hands on the thighs.

7.   Lift the crown of the head and lengthen the spine upward. Keep the knees and ankles relaxed.

Hold this pose for several deep breaths or the duration of your meditation practice. Inhale, lengthening the spine. Exhale, allowing the knees to sink lower.

*This variation of **Swastikasana** is especially suitable for beginners working on pelvic alignment and straightening the spine. Elevating the hands on blocks also promotes chest opening, allowing for deeper breathing in this pose.*

Swastikasana with a strap

Relief of the knees

1.   Get into *Swastikasana* (p. 131).

2.   Place a strap around the knees.

3.   Tighten the strap to support the legs' weight and relax the knees.

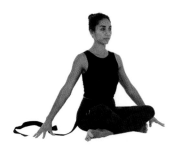

Hold this pose for several deep breaths or the duration of your meditation practice. Inhale, lengthening the spine. Exhale, allowing the knees to sink lower.

Especially at the beginning of the practice, sitting in meditation for a long time can feel quite challenging. This variation helps beginners to achieve a more relaxed meditation posture. The strap supports the weight of the legs, relieving the knee joints and lower back.

Swastikasana with a bolster and a blanket

Pelvic alignment/relief of the lower back

1.   Sit on a bolster aligned lengthwise with the mat.

2.   Assume *Swastikasana* (p. 131).

3.   Roll a blanket between the knees and shins.

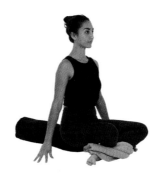

Stay in this pose for a few breaths or the duration of your meditation practice.

Beginners often find crossing the shins uncomfortable. The support of the blanket reduces pressure, allowing the lymph nodes to relax.

Gomukhasana—Cow Face

Go = cow, *Mukha* = face

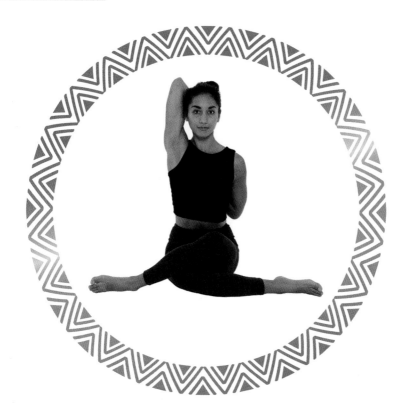

Gomukhasana, or Cow Face, is one of yoga's most complex seated postures. It opens both the shoulders and hips. Stretching the deep hip muscles can alleviate lower back pain. Chest expansion encourages deep breathing and aims to relax the shoulder muscles.

Energetically, it stimulates the root, sacral, and heart chakras. Due to the unfamiliar physical position, *Gomukhasana* also impacts mental flexibility. Thoughts may calm down, and emotional blockages, believed in yoga to reside in the hips, can be released.

Avoid this pose if you have chronic or acute knee issues.

Gomukhasana with a block and a strap

Pelvic alignment/relief of the knees/shoulder opening

1. Begin by sitting on a flat block with the strap within easy reach.

2. Extend your right leg forward and bend your left leg, crossing the thigh over the right leg.

3. Bend your right leg as well, stacking the knees. Place your feet on the sides of the block and roll your calves outward to align the pelvis.

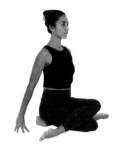

4. Grab the strap with your right hand and lift the arm overhead, keeping it close to your ear. Allow the long end of the strap to hang down.

5. Stretch your left arm to the side, tilting the shoulder forward so that the back of the hand faces forward.

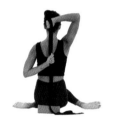

6. Bend your left arm and with your left hand reach for the long end of the strap behind your back.

7. Bring your hands closer together and pull on both ends of the strap. Straighten your spine.

8. Inhale into the chest, further elongating the spine. Exhale into the abdomen, allowing the pelvis to sink heavier onto the block.

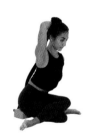

Stay in this pose for several deep breaths.

Using props is crucial, especially for beginners. The block's elevation helps with pelvic alignment and knee stacking when hip flexibility is limited.

The strap enables a more open chest and extended spine, particularly useful if the shoulders aren't flexible enough to clasp the hands behind the back as in the regular pose.

Paschimottanasana—Seated Forward Bend

Pashchim = entire body, *Ut* = intensive, *Tan* = stretch

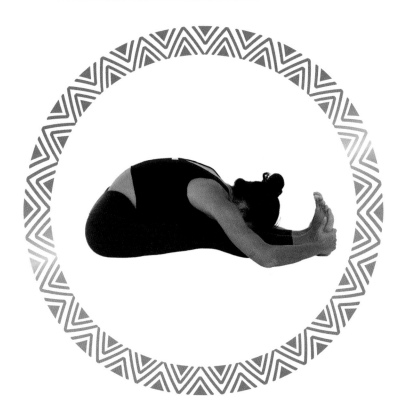

Paschimottanasana is one of the most important and intense Forward Bends in Hatha Yoga. Stretching the entire spine allows the breath to flow through the back ribs to the upper back, influencing the function of the kidneys, bladder, and pancreas.

Bending the head forward relieves the cervical spine and affects the respiratory center. The heart receives a gentle massage, and the liver and digestive organs are stimulated. Energetically, *Paschimottanasana* stimulates the root chakra and the third eye chakra through deep bowing and introspective posture.

Paschimottanasana with a blanket

Alignment of the pelvis/support for the lower back

1.   Sit on the front edge of a carefully folded blanket.

2.   Extend your legs in front of you. Flex your feet and slightly open your hips.

3.   Align yourself over the midpoint of both sit bones, and keep the lower back long.

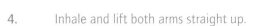

4.   Inhale and lift both arms straight up.

5.   Exhale and hinge forward from the hips, gently drawing the lower abdomen inward and upward. Keep the lower back long and the legs active.

6.   Rest the upper body on your thighs, or as near your thighs as you can reach. Place your arms beside your legs or reach for the outer edges of your feet. Relax the shoulders.

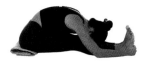

Stay for several deep breaths in this pose. Without losing length in the lower back, allow the upper back to round and sink deeper into the Forward Bend. Slowly roll up to release the pose.

To maintain length in the lower back, pelvic alignment is crucial. The elevation through the blanket prevents the buttocks from lifting off the floor and the foundation of the pose from shifting.

Paschimottanasana with a strap

Stretching the back of the legs/spinal stretch

1.   Come into an upright seated position.

2.   Bend your legs and place a strap around the soles of your feet. Feet are flexed.

3.   Hold one end of the strap in each hand, rolling the shoulders back and pushing the chest forward.

4.   Slowly start sliding your feet into the strap to straighten your legs.

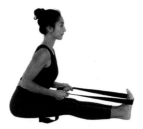

Stay in this pose for several deep breaths. Keep the strap taut while keeping the shoulders as relaxed as possible.

Pulling on the strap helps to lengthen the spine from the hips. The thighs are activated, protecting the hamstrings in their intense stretch.

Paschimottanasana with a strap

Pelvic alignment/activation of the outer thighs

1. Begin by sitting upright, placing a strap at the level of your sacrum. Bend your legs and position the balls of your feet in the wide loop of the strap.

2. Place your palms beside your hips and slowly start straightening your legs.

3. Inhale as you lift your chest forward, lengthening the spine. Keep the strap taut.

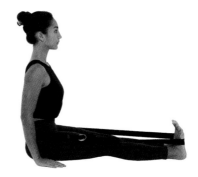

Stay in this pose for several deep breaths.

This variation helps align the pelvis and serves as preparation for the full Forward Bend. It stretches both the hamstrings and maintains length in the lower back.

Paschimottanasana with a block

Intense stretching of the back of the legs

1. Place a block flat at the end of your mat. Sit upright in front of the block.

2. Extend your legs forward and place your heels on the block.

3. Flex your feet and actively press your heels into the block.

4. Inhale deeply as you reach your arms up, lengthening the spine.

5. Exhale and reach for the outer edges of your feet. Alternatively, you can use a strap for assistance.

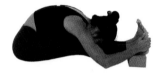

Stay in this pose for several deep breaths.

This variation is ideal for advanced practitioners seeking to deepen the intensity of the pose. Elevating the heels activates the back of the legs, intensifying the stretch in the calves, hamstrings, and Achilles tendons. It also strengthens the thigh muscles, providing additional support for the knees.

Paschimottanasana with a block

Intense stretch of the back of the legs/elongating the lower back

1.   Begin by placing a block lengthwise at the end of your mat.

2.   Sitting upright, extend your legs in front of you, pressing the soles of your feet against the block.

3.   Inhale deeply as you reach your arms up, lengthening the spine.

4.   Exhale and hinge forward from the hips, gripping the outer edges of the block with both hands.

5.   Actively press the soles of your feet into the block as you extend the lower back and deepen into the Forward Bend.

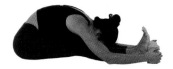

Stay in this pose for several deep breaths.

The block acts as an extension of the legs, which is particularly beneficial for flexible practitioners or those with long arms, intensifying the stretch in the back of the legs. Actively holding the block also aids in better elongation of the lower back.

Pressing the soles into the block activates the thigh muscles, protecting the knees during leg extension.

Janu Sirsasana—Head-Knee Pose

Janu = knee, *Sirsha* = head

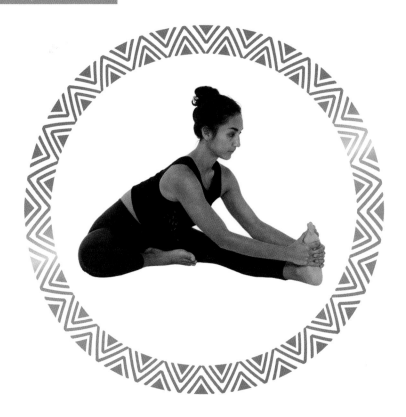

In this pose, the entire posterior chain receives a deep stretch. The initial hip opening facilitates greater extension of the lower back, leading to a profound stretch along the spine, shoulders, groin, and back of the legs.

The breath flows into the back flanks, stimulating energy flow to the adrenal glands. The elongation of the back naturally propels the chest forward, activating the heart chakra.

Janu Sirsasana with a blanket and a strap

Pelvic alignment/support of the back

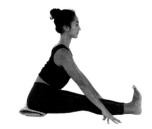

1. Sit on the front edge of a carefully folded blanket.

2. Bend the left leg and place the sole of the foot on the inside of the right thigh.

3. Flex the left foot and actively push it to the inside of the right leg. Feel the pelvis lifting.

Optional:

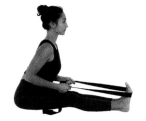

4. Place a strap around the right foot. Grip the ends of the strap with both hands.

5. Inhale, lift the chest, and lengthen the entire spine.

6. Exhale and slide the right foot into the strap to straighten the leg.

Keep the back long and bend deeper into the Forward Bend over the thighs. Stay in this pose for several deep breaths. Slowly rise and switch to the other side.

The elevation provided by the blanket helps beginners to align the pelvis better and extend the spine forward. The strap also assists yogis with very long legs to sink deeper into the Forward Bend without curving the back.

Janu Sirsasana with a bolster

Alignment of the bent leg/hip opening

1. Place a bolster horizontally across the mat.

2. Sit with the left buttock positioned on the outer edge of the bolster, extending the left leg straight in front of you.

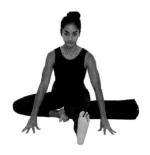

3. Bend the right leg and rest the sole of the foot on the bolster, ensuring the knee forms a right angle with the front leg and aligns with the bolster.

4. Inhale deeply, extending the arms overhead to elongate the entire spine.

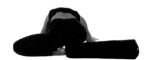

5. Exhale slowly, maintaining a long back as you hinge forward from the hips. Reach for the outer edge of the foot and deepen into the Forward Bend.

Remain in this posture for several deep breaths. Then, gradually rise and switch sides.

---

*In the traditional variation of **Janu Sirsasana**, the hips are opened at a right angle. Using the bolster for elevation facilitates proper alignment of the bent leg, thereby enhancing the stretch along the front of the thigh during the Forward Bend.*

Janu Sirsasana with a block

Activation of the thigh/stretching the back of the leg

1. Begin by placing a block upright at the end of your mat, then move into an upright seated position.

2. Extend your left leg long in front of you and lean the sole of your foot against the block.

3. Bend your right leg and place the sole of your foot on the inside of your left thigh, allowing the knee to lower toward the mat gently.

4. As you inhale, raise your arms overhead, extending and stretching the entire spine.

5. Exhale and maintain a long back as you hinge forward from the hips. Hold onto the outer edges of the block.

6. Firmly grip the block with both hands, rolling your shoulder blades back and extending your chest toward the block.

7. Slide the sole of your foot into the block and engage your thigh muscles. Sink deeper into the Forward Bend.

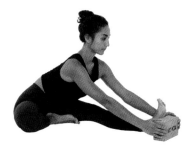

Take several deep breaths in this pose before switching sides.

The block acts as an extension of the extended leg, assisting those with a longer torso to deepen their Forward Bend. This variation intensifies the stretch, and sliding the foot into the block activates the thigh muscles for a more effective stretch.

Virasana—Hero Pose

Vira = hero

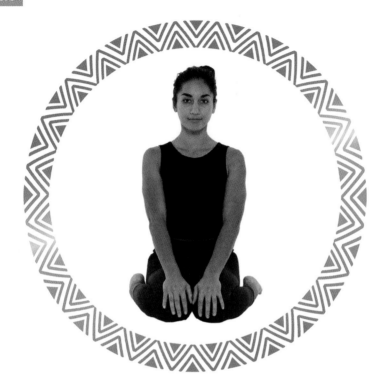

Hero Pose is an intense seated posture used in Hatha Yoga as an alternative meditation seat or for Pranayama (breath techniques). The posture promotes circulation in the knee and hip joints, as well as the large muscle groups of the legs, especially the quadriceps. It progressively loosens stiff hips and maintains flexibility in ankles and knees.

Avoid this pose if there's an injury or prior strain in the knees or ankles. A gentler variation is *Adha Virasana*, where only one leg is bent. Mentally, Hero Pose might pose an initial challenge.

But once overcome, it stands for mental clarity and immediately feels invigorating. Energetically, it mainly addresses the root and sacral chakras.

By aligning the spine in *Virasana*, the yogi can navigate through all energy centers with the help of the breath.

Virasana with a bolster

Pelvic alignment/relief for knees and lower back

1. Place a bolster lengthwise on your mat.

2. Sit on the bolster and extend your legs backward. The shins are on the floor, and the feet rest on the sides of the bolster with toes pointing back.

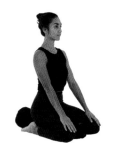

3. Roll the calves outward, letting both ischial bones sink deep into the bolster. The outer thighs touch the inner sides of the calves.

4. Align the spine and rest your hands on the thighs. Shoulders are relaxed.

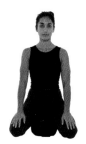

Stay in this pose for a few deep breaths. You can close your eyes and linger in meditation.

*This variation offers a gentle alternative to **Hero Pose**, suitable for those with less open hips, providing relief to the knees. The elevated seating on the bolster helps beginners lift the pelvis and elongate the spine.*

Virasana with a block and a blanket

Pelvic alignment/relief for the ankle joints

1.   Sit on a block.

2.   Extend your legs back into *Virasana*. Place a rolled blanket under the tops of your feet.

3.   Align the pelvis over the block and elongate the entire spine. Rest your hands on your thighs. Shoulders are relaxed.

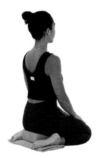

Stay in this pose for a few deep breaths. You may close your eyes and meditate.

The elevated seat aids pelvic alignment while supporting the lower back, and the blanket relieves pressure on the ankles. This variation is particularly suitable for those with sensitive feet or knees.

Balasana—Child's Pose

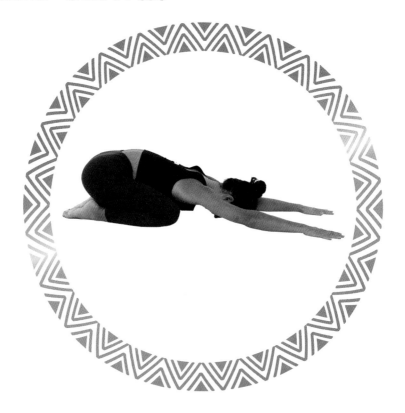

Balasana is one of the less physically demanding poses, but it brings many body-positive benefits for system harmonization. The pose's physical form triggers our early childhood memory, positively affecting the nervous system. The connection between the abdomen and thighs makes the breath rhythm palpable, acting as a massage for abdominal organs, particularly influencing digestion.

Hips, thighs, ankles, and spine are gently stretched, promoting circulation. Child's Pose is a soothing relief, especially for lower back discomfort. The sinking into the hips primarily stimulates the root and sacral chakras. The forward-bending posture directs breath to the back of the body, boosting energy flow to the back of the heart chakra.

The gentle placement of the forehead on the ground focuses the mind on the third eye, considered a gateway to inner wisdom. *Balasana* turns attention inward, allowing the yogi mental introspection.

Balasana with a block

Pelvic support/relief of the knees

1. Sit on a flat block in a kneeling position.

2. Open your knees wide enough for your hands to comfortably move forward.

3. Extend your arms forward, placing your forehead on the ground.

4. Inhale and elongate the spine forward. Exhale and lower the pelvis back toward the heels.

5. Relax your forearms onto the ground, keeping the shoulders away from the ears.

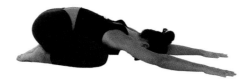

Stay in this pose for a few deep breaths. Place your hands under your shoulders and, supported by your arms, roll back into an upright seat.

The block's support aids beginners in achieving the posture, especially when the hips aren't open enough to comfortably rest the buttocks on the heels. The elevation reduces tension in the thighs, providing relief for the knees.

Balasana with a strap and two blocks

Spinal stretch/chest opening

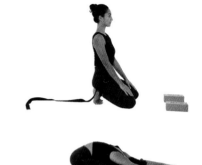

1. Place two flat blocks shoulder width apart at the front of the mat.

2. Come into an upright kneeling pose and secure a strap around both thighs and ankles.

3. Lean forward, placing your palms on the blocks. Keep the hips resting on the heels.

4. Slide the blocks forward to extend the arms and intensify the stretch in the sides of the body. Place your forehead on the ground.

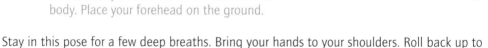

Stay in this pose for a few deep breaths. Bring your hands to your shoulders. Roll back up to a seated position, using your arms as a support.

This variation offers advanced practitioners the opportunity to enhance spinal elongation. The strap helps to anchor the pelvis, allowing the lower back and the rest of the spine to extend further. Elevating the forearms with the blocks opens the chest more, intensifying the stretch in the sides.

Supta Padangusthasana—Reclining Hand-To-Big-Toe Pose

Supta = lie down, *Pada* = feet, *Angushta* = big toe

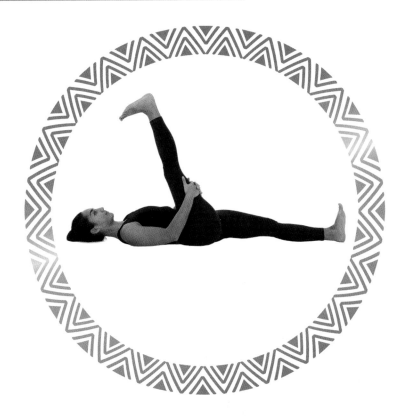

In this intense reclined leg stretch, relief is offered as the back of the leg is stretched, promoting pelvic mobility. The prone position enhances blood circulation in the legs. Maintaining proper pelvic alignment in the posture has a soothing effect on the lower back.

It stretches and strengthens the knee and calf muscles, hip joints, and lumbar spine. *Supta Padangusthasana* can also be beneficial for relieving sciatic pain and menstrual discomfort in the lower back.

Energetically, pelvic alignment holds significance for the root chakra. The posture has a simultaneously uplifting and stimulating effect on the mind.

Supta Padangusthasana with a strap

Pelvic alignment/relief of the shoulders

1. Lie on your back, ensuring you have a strap within reach.

2. Bring your right knee toward your chest using both hands while the left leg remains extended on the ground with the foot flexed and the heel touching the floor.

3. Place the strap around the sole of your right foot.

4. Hold both ends of the strap close to your body, keeping your shoulders relaxed.

5. Slowly slide your right foot further into the strap and begin straightening the leg.

6. Press the left heel firmly into the mat as you engage both legs with flexed feet, activating the muscles of the thighs.

7. Inhale as you lengthen the right leg, feeling the opening in the back of the leg.

8. Exhale and focus on grounding the right buttock, ensuring closed hips with the toes of the right foot pointing straight toward your body.

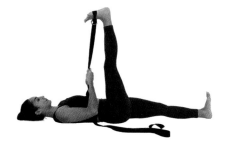

Remain in *Supta Padangusthasana* for several deep breaths, then slowly bend the right leg and release the strap. Repeat the sequence on the other side.

The strap acts as an extension of your arms, allowing for relaxed shoulders and requiring minimal arm strength. Additionally, it assists both beginners and advanced practitioners in aligning the pelvis, thereby enhancing the stretch in the back of the leg and lengthening the lower back.

Variation 1 for Supta Padangusthasana with a strap

Hip opening

1. Come into variation 1 for *Supta Padangusthasana* with a strap.

2. Hold both ends of the strap with the right hand, releasing the left hand.

3. Slowly lower the right leg to the side, keeping the left buttock on the ground.

4. Place the left hand on the left thigh to prevent lifting the hip.

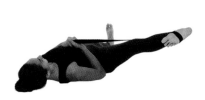

Stay for several deep breaths in the hip-opening position. Slowly bring the leg back to the center, bend the leg, and release the strap. Repeat everything on the other side.

The resistance of the strap allows the extended leg to be lowered toward the mat slowly and in a controlled manner. this keeps the inner thighs engaged and the pelvis in its correct alignment.

Twist Variation 2: Parivrtta Supta Padangusthasana with a strap

Spinal twist

1. After practicing variation 2 of *Supta Padangusthasana* with a strap, return to variation 1.

2. Transfer both ends of the strap to the left hand, and extend the right arm to shoulder height beside you.

3. Slide the inner side of the right foot into the strap and gradually lower the right leg to the left side.

4. Ensure the right shoulder blade remains grounded while the left leg stays actively extended with the foot flexed and the heel pressing into the mat.

5. Guide the right leg to the left side, experiencing the stretch along the outer side of the right thigh. Internally rotate the hip of the right leg while keeping the left hip straight.

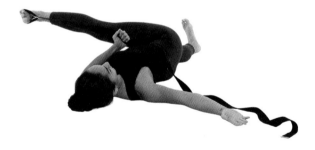

Remain in this pose for several deep breaths. Slowly bring the leg back to the center with strength and control, then release the strap. Repeat the sequence (including variations 1, 2, and 3) on the other side.

In the twisted variation of **Supta Padangusthasana**, the spine experiences an intense stretch and twist. This stretches the lower back, especially the quadratus lumborum muscle and the iliotibial band on the outer side of the thigh.

The twist helps to release blockages in the chest and, especially, the lumbar spine, reducing tension in the abdomen. This has beneficial effects on digestion and spinal flexibility.

All lying variations of **Padangusthasana** prepare the alignment of the pelvis for standing balance poses.

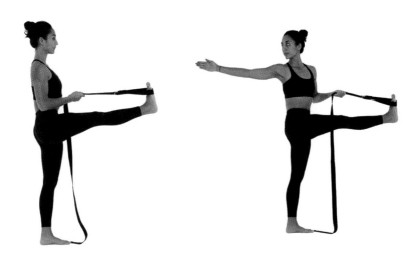

6
RELAXATION
Restorative Yoga
& Yin Yoga

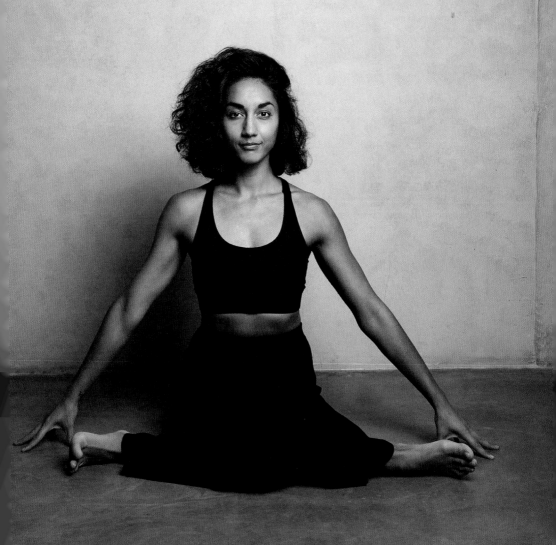

Supta Baddha Konasana—Reclining Butterfly

Supta = reclined, *Baddha* = bound, *Kona* = angle

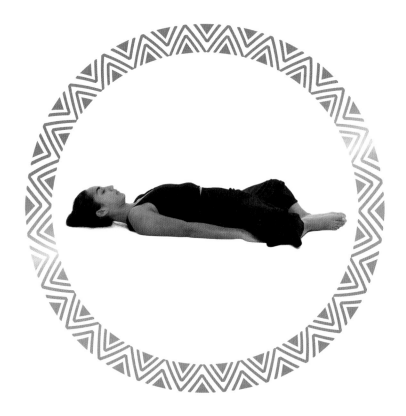

The Supine Bound Angle Pose is another term for the *Reclining Butterfly*. The knees descend like two open wings to the sides. Due to gravity, the thighs and inner legs stretch without muscular support, opening the groin.

The passive hip opening targets the sacral chakra and stimulates the reproductive organs. Additionally, the abdomen can relax, initiating digestive processes. This pose may act as a spasm-relieving and pain-reducing remedy for menstrual discomfort.

Supta Baddha Konasana with a bolster

Gentle hip opening/relief of the lower back

1.   Place a bolster horizontally across the center of the mat.

2.   Sit upright, facing toward the bolster. Place your feet over the bolster.

3.   Grasp your thighs with both hands, slowly rolling down onto your back.

4.   Bring the soles of your feet together, letting the knees fall to the sides. The outer thighs relax in contact with the bolster.

5.   Place the backs of your hands on the mat beside your body. Close your eyes. With each deep exhale, let your legs sink heavier into the bolster.

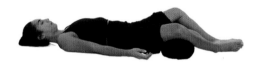

*This passive variation of **Supta Baddha Konasana** promotes overall rejuvenation. The body releases muscular tension, allowing the breath to flow freely. This brings the organs and mind into a deeply relaxed state.*

Supta Baddha Konasana with a bolster and two blocks

Gentle hip opening/relief of the knees/passive heart opening

1. Lay the bolster lengthwise in the center of your mat. Keep two blocks handy.

2. Lie down on the bolster, letting your spine rest on it.

3. Allow your knees to drop to the sides.

4. Slide the blocks under the outer sides of your thighs.

5. Place your hands beside your body, palms facing up.

6. Close your eyes, take deep breaths into the chest, and let the back sink into the support with each exhale.

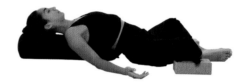

*This variation of **Supta Baddha Konasana** is suitable for anyone looking to indulge in the regenerative effects on the front of the body. You can fully release your body weight onto the bolster; the blocks support sensitive knee joints.*

Supta Baddha Konasana with a block

Intensive hip opening

1. Lie on your back. Have a block within reach. Place your feet hip width apart.

2. Lift your hips and slide a flat block under your pelvis.

3. Rest your sacrum on the block. Bring your feet together and close your knees.

4. Slowly, let your knees drop to the sides.

5. Slide your hands under your thighs. Release tension in your groins with each exhale.

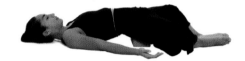

As you progress, you can free your hands from under the thighs, letting gravity enhance the hip opening.

This variation is intense and particularly targets hip flexibility. Avoid it if you have lower back issues.

Matsyasana—Supported Backbend

Matsya = fish

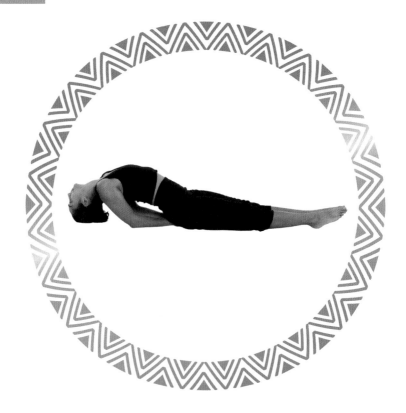

*Matsyasana—or fish pose—*is a heart-opening Backbend that can benefit from props and support. It helps release tension in the shoulder and back muscles. Opening the chest allows for deeper breaths, revitalizing the mind and combating lethargy.

Emotionally, *Matsyasana* mainly addresses blockages in the heart chakra, fostering feelings of joy and openness.

Matsyasana with a blanket

Gentle heart opening/shoulder relief

1. Roll a blanket and place it horizontally across the center of your mat.

2. Sit upright with your back to the blanket, soles of the feet planted on the mat.

3. Slowly rolling down and back, rest on the rolled blanket. Lower your chin to your chest, keeping your neck long.

4. Extend your arms over the body, ensuring your shoulders are away from your ears.

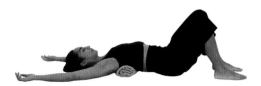

5. To enhance the stretch in the front of your body, you can stretch your legs out in front. If you have lower back discomfort, keep your feet planted on the mat.

6. Close your eyes and breathe deeply into the chest. With each inhale, expand the ribcage; with each exhale, let the chest sink deeper into the blanket.

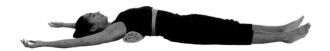

Stay in the pose for up to 5 minutes. To release, bring your feet back and slowly turn to the side, legs drawn in. Take a moment to feel the effects of the pose before sitting upright.

The rolled blanket elevates the chest into a profound heart opening, allowing the body's weight to be fully released. Shoulders and neck are relieved.

Matsyasana with a bolster

Passive heart opening/upper body relief

1. Place a bolster lengthwise in the center of your mat.

2. Sit with your back just in front of the edge of the bolster—feet planted on the ground.

3. Slowly lower your spine onto the bolster.

4. To fully relax, you can extend your legs forward. If you have lower back issues, keep your feet planted on the floor.

5. Close your eyes and breathe deeply into the front of your body. Feel your heart rise with each inhale. With each exhale, let the weight of your upper body sink deeper into the bolster.

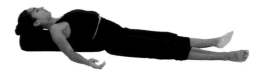

You can stay in this pose for up to 15 minutes. To release, grab your thighs with both hands, tuck your chin to your chest, and roll up to a seated position, rounding your upper back forward for a moment.

The bolster provides gentle support for the spine, allowing the front of the body to open. You can fully surrender the weight of your torso, letting your entire body relax in this pose.

Matsyasana with a block

Passive Backbend/upper back relief

1. Place a flat block horizontally in the center of your mat.

2. Sit with your back facing the block, and feet planted on the ground.

3. Grab your knees with both hands. Slowly roll back, resting the back of your chest on the block. Lower your chin to your chest, keeping your neck long. If this is uncomfortable, place a folded blanket under your head.

4. Extend your arms over the body, shoulders away from the ears. You can stay here or:

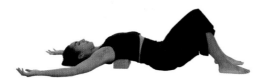

5. Stretch your legs. Bring your feet back up if it feels uncomfortable in the lower back.

6. Close your eyes and breathe deeply into the chest. With each inhale, expand the ribcage. With each exhale, let the chest sink deeper into the block.

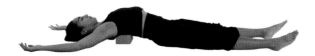

Stay in this pose for up to 2 minutes. To release, grab your thighs with both hands, tuck your chin to your chest, and roll up to a seated position, rounding your upper back forward for a moment.

The elevation from the block provides a platform for a passive Backbend and heart opening. You can fully release the weight of your torso, relieving the head, neck, and shoulders.

Jathara Parivartanasana—Lying Twist

Jathara = abdomen, *Parivarasana* = move back and forth

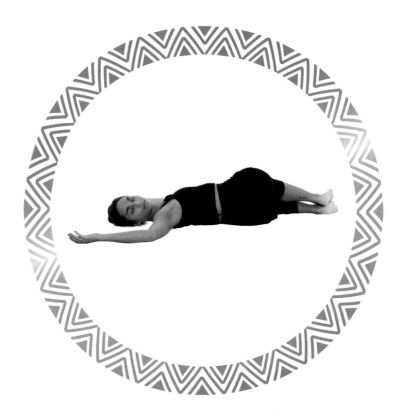

Even though the back is completely relaxed, the lying twist keeps the spine mobile. Opening the sides of the body stretches the intercostal muscles between the ribs and promotes deep breathing. The mind can relax. The gentle twist massages the organs in the abdominal area.

This has a digestive effect and energetically affects the solar plexus and heart chakras. In cases of chronic and acute discomfort in the lower back, the twist should only be performed with props, if at all.

Jathara Parivartanasana with a bolster

Relief for the lower back

1.   Come to lying on your back. Keep a bolster handy next to you. Place your feet in the middle of the mat, with the insides touching.

2.   Extend your arms at a right angle at shoulder height. Anchor your shoulder blades firmly into the mat.

3.   Lift your pelvis and swing your hips to the right. Place the pelvis on the right side and let the knees sink to the left.

4.   Place the bolster between the insides of the legs.

5.   If your neck allows, turn your head in the opposite direction. Lower your chin to your chest.

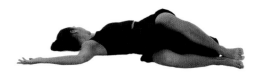

Stay in this pose for up to 3 minutes. Breathe deeply between your chest and abdomen. First, turn your head back. Then, bring your pelvis back to the center and switch to the other side.

The bolster releases tension in the lower back and relieves the lumbar spine and shoulders.

Jathara Parivartanasana with a block

Relief for the lower back/relief for the shoulders

1. Place a flat block horizontally on the left side of the mat.

2. Lie on your back. Feet are planted on the floor. The insides of the legs touch at the center of the mat.

3. Extend your arms at a right angle at shoulder height. Anchor your shoulder blades firmly into the mat.

4. Lift your legs at a right angle to the body and let the knees sink to the block on the right.

5. If your neck allows, turn your head in the opposite direction. Lower your chin to your chest.

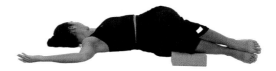

Stay in this pose for several deep breaths. With each inhale, feel the opening of the shoulders. With each exhale, let the legs sink heavier into the block. First, turn your head back. Then, bring the legs back to the center and switch to the other side.

For additional relief, you can place a rolled blanket between the knees.

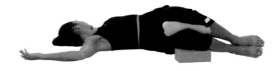

The block allows for precise alignment of the legs at a right angle to the body, providing optimal stretching for the back and shoulders.

Balasana—Child's Pose

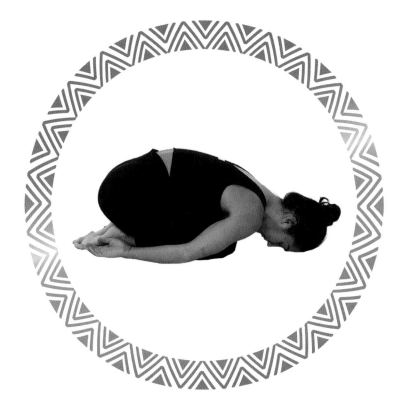

As described on page 150, the Child's Pose has a very calming effect on the nervous system. The curled-up position, resembling an embryo in the uterus, signals the brain a sense of protection and safety. Deep breathing supports this sensation. Contact between the abdomen and thighs allows the heartbeat from the abdominal aorta to be felt directly (it is transmitted through the intestine in front of it).

Deep belly breathing calms the parasympathetic nervous system, stimulates bowel activity through the pressure of the thighs, and contributes to overall relaxation. The spine experiences a gentle stretch, freeing up energy flow to the kidneys by opening the surrounding fascial structures.

The root and sacral chakras are engaged by sinking back into the hips and grounding the pelvis. In the withdrawal of the pose, we can focus on inner wisdom—letting go of external events.

Balasana with a bolster

Relief for the lower back and neck

1.   Place a bolster lengthwise in the center of the mat.

2.   Kneel in front of the bolster and open your knees mat width apart.

3.   Cross your forearms and rest your forehead on them, gripping with both hands.

4.   Relax your upper body into the bolster.

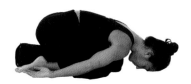

Stay in this pose for up to 5 minutes, breathing deeply into your abdomen.

*In this variation of **Balasana**, the torso's weight can be fully supported by the bolster, relieving the lower back. Resting the head on the elevation reduces pressure on the cervical spine. The neck can relax.*

Balasana with a bolster and a block

Relief for the torso

1. Place a flat block at the front of the mat. Place the short end of the bolster on the block so that the head end is slightly elevated. The other end of the bolster rests in the center of the mat.

2. Kneel in front of the bolster and open your knees mat width apart. Lower your upper body onto the bolster.

3. Shift your hips back toward your heels while hugging the bolster. Place your arms behind your body and rest the backs of your hands on the mat.

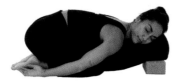

Stay in this pose for 1–2 minutes. Breathe deeply into your abdomen. Then, turn your head to the other side before you sit back up.

*In this variation of **Balasana**, the entire weight of the torso can rest on the bolster. The pelvis can sink deeper back and relax between the hips. This provides particularly soothing relief for the lower back.*

Anahatasana—Melting Heart Pose

Anahata = heart

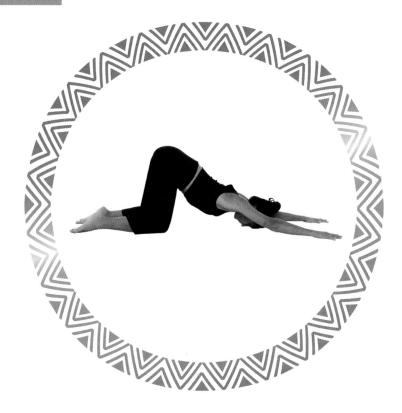

Also known as *Uttana Shishosana*, translated as Puppy Pose, *Anahatasana* directs attention to the heart area. In this modified version of Downward Facing Dog, the upper back is stretched, the shoulder girdle and chest are opened, and the heart chakra is stimulated.

Anahatasana with a block

Relief of the cervical spine

1.   Place a flat block horizontally in the center of your mat.

2.   Come into Tabletop position, then walk your arms forward, resting your forehead on the block.

3.   Press your hands into the ground and keep your arms active. Keep your buttocks above your knees and the tops of your feet resting on the mat.

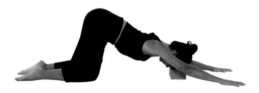

Stay in the pose for several deep breaths. Keep your arms active without lifting your shoulders to your ears. Your neck should be relaxed. If you have knee problems, you can place a blanket under your knees.

Resting your forehead on the block reduces pressure on the cervical spine and makes it easier to move your shoulder blades back. This allows for further opening of the chest and expansion of the breathing spaces.

Anahatasana with a bolster

Relieve shoulder tension/intense chest stretch

1.   Place a bolster horizontally at the front of your mat.

2.   Move into Tabletop position. Extend your arms forward and rest your forehead on
        the bolster.

3.   Bend your arms and bring your palms together. Lower your thumbs toward your
        shoulder blades.

4.   Breathe deeply into the stretch of the chest. Keep your buttocks above your knees
        and the tops of your feet resting on the mat.

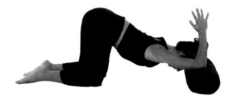

Stay here for several deep breaths. Keep your neck relaxed. You can place a blanket under
your knees if you have knee issues.

*The elevation provided by the bolster makes it easier to relax into the heart opening of the
pose. As the name **Melting Heart** suggests, you may allow the chest to broaden further and
melt deeper toward the mat. In this arm variation, the upper arms are stretched, and the sides
are stretched more intensely.*

Upavistha Konasana—Wide-Angle Seated Forward Bend

Upavishta = seated, *Kona* = angle

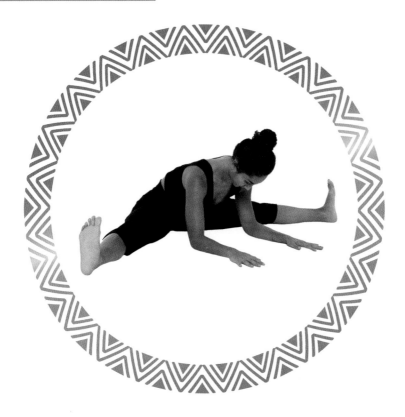

As page 127 describes, *Upavistha Konasana* is one of the seated hip openers. In the passive variation, the upper body is folded forward, extending the pose into a Forward Bend, stretching the inner thighs, hips, and back of the body.

By sinking into this hip-opening Forward Bend, the mind can relax, and emotional blockages stored as tension patterns in the tissue can be released.

Wide-Angle Seated Forward Bend is particularly suitable for pregnant women or for relieving menstrual discomfort. It opens the pelvis, stimulates the pelvic floor and digestive organs, and, when combined with the Forward Bend, has a calming effect on the nervous system.

Upavistha Konasana with a bolster and a block

Relief to the upper body and the neck

1.   Place an upright block at the front of your mat. Lay the bolster with the head end on the block and the other end of the mat.

2.   Sit in a wide-leg straddle. Your legs frame the bolster and the block. Keep your feet flexed.

3.   Rest your forehead on the bolster. Keep your pelvis upright. If this is challenging, you can also place a folded blanket under your buttocks. Let your arms rest relaxed beside your body.

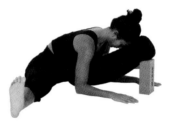

Stay in this pose for up to 5 minutes. Breathe deeply into the back of your body. With each exhale, sink further into the Forward Bend.

The bolster allows the upper body to relax forward. Instead of actively stretching, let the muscles gradually relax in the desired direction.

Upavistha Konasana against the wall

Passive stretch to the inner thighs/hip opening

1. Sit sideways next to a wall, leaving about a fist-width distance between you and the wall.

2. Bring one extended leg at a time against the wall and lower your upper body to the floor. Your gaze is now directed toward your feet.

3. Slowly, let your extended legs sink toward the sides. Keep your feet flexed and heels resting against the wall.

4. Rest your hands on your legs and breathe deeply into the wide straddle.

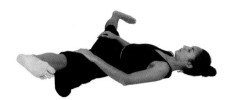

Breathe deeply into the stretch and stay in this pose for up to a minute. For support, you can place a blanket or a flat block under your buttocks. Before turning onto your side, put your feet flat against the wall.

Leaning against the wall allows you to relax into a deep hip opening.

Viparita Karani—Supported Shoulder Stand

Viparita = reverse , *Karani* = form

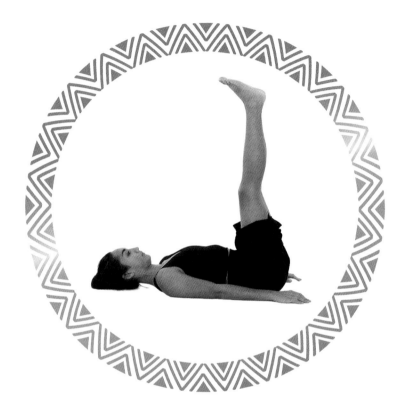

Unlike the Shoulder Stand (p.110), Viparita Karani places no strain on the shoulders and cervical spine. The Supported Shoulder Stand serves as a refreshing pause for the system, significantly rejuvenating the legs and promoting overall benefits for the nervous system.

Elevating the legs directly in the line of gravity increases the return of oxygen-depleted blood to the body's center. This proves advantageous for regenerating and eliminating acidic metabolic by-products from the pelvis and lower extremities in a healthy cardiovascular system.

The passive inversion pose, particularly beneficial for a stressed system, imparts a soothing effect. However, it is not advisable for individuals with elevated eye pressure, high blood pressure, hyperthyroidism, or inflammation in the head area.

Viparita Karani against the wall/optionally with a bolster

Relief of the legs/relief of the lower back

1.   Begin by sitting sideways with a hand-width distance from the wall, keeping your legs bent and your spine upright.

2.   Twist your torso away from the wall, bringing the soles of your feet to rest against it.

3.   Adjust your legs to form a right angle above the pelvis, ensuring that your upper body is aligned straight toward the wall.

4.   Gradually straighten your legs, allowing your heels to rest comfortably on the wall.

5.   Position your hands beside your body or on your abdomen.

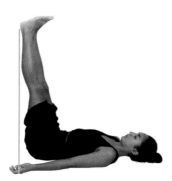

Remain in this posture for up to 2 minutes. Gently draw your knees toward your chest one by one, then transition onto your side with your legs pulled up. Lay on your side and feel the effect of the pose for a few moments before slowly sitting up.

*This variation of **Viparita Karani** is an excellent choice for relieving lower back discomfort. With the support of the wall, the lumbar spine experiences complete relief. The legs no longer bear weight, resulting in the release of tension and heaviness.*

Viparita Karani with a block (or a bolster)

Intensifying the pose

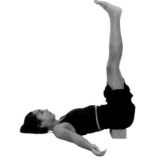

1. Lie on your back, keeping a block nearby.

2. Place your feet hip width apart and lift your hips, sliding the block under your buttocks.

Stay in this **Supported Shoulder Stand** variation if lifting your legs feels too intense.

3. Lower your sacrum onto the block and slowly lift your legs, one at a time.

4. Let your legs hover over your pelvis, with your arms resting beside your body.

Stay in this pose for up to a minute. Then, slowly lower your feet back down, lift your hips, and move the block aside. Bring both knees to your chest to relieve the lower back.

This variation is suitable for yogis who want to enhance the energetic effects of the inversion without muscular exertion. The block elevates the pelvis onto a pedestal, influencing the energetic impact on the root chakra.

Optionally, you can place a bolster under the pelvis instead of the block.

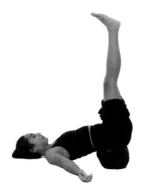

Shavasana—Corpse Pose

Shava = corpse

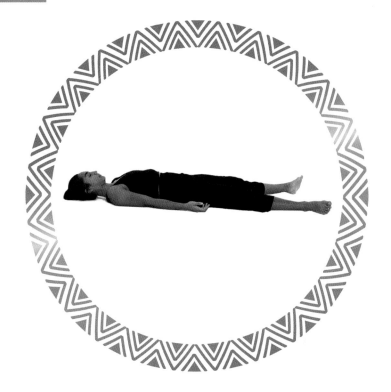

Shavasana, commonly known as the final relaxation pose in the physical yoga practice, is one of the most popular poses. The body can completely relax after stimulating the system through movement and breath. Muscles, bones, and the entire body weight surrender to gravity.

The senses withdraw, creating a sense of unity. Neither mind nor body are now distracted by externalities. Iyengar refers to *Shavasana* as the first step into meditation.

In relaxation, the rhythm of breath and heartbeat slows down, blood pressure decreases, and the moment of regeneration can set in. Although *Shavasana* is the most restful of all yoga poses, it is not always easy initially, as mental restlessness and physical discomfort may manifest here.

The use of props, however, can help make the pose even more relaxing.

Shavasana with a bolster

Relief of the lower back

1. Place a bolster horizontally in the center of your mat. Sit up straight, facing toward the bolster.

2. Position your feet over the bolster.

3. With both hands, grip your thighs and roll down to lie on your back.

4. Allow the backs of your knees to rest on the bolster, and let your legs slide forward.

5. Place the backs of your hands beside your body, letting your fingers sink outward. Relax your shoulder blades onto the mat.

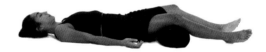

Remain in this pose for up to 15 minutes. Your body can fully unwind, and you can release the weight of your legs onto the bolster.

Using the bolster helps the large thigh muscles relax, while elevating the legs relieves the lower back, which remains flat on the ground.

Shavasana with a bolster

Relief of the lower back

1. Come into *Shavasana*, ensuring you have a bolster with handles nearby.

2. Position the bolster horizontally in the pelvic area.

3. Allow the backs of your hands to rest beside your body, with your fingers gently spreading outward and your shoulder blades relaxed on the mat.

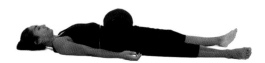

Remain in this pose for up to 15 minutes.

The added weight of the bolster deepens your connection to the ground, allowing your lower back to softly meld into the mat, elongating the spine. This variation is especially beneficial following a yoga session with vigorous Backbends.

Shavasana in the prone position with a bolster

Relief for the upper and lower back

1. Position a bolster lengthwise in the center of your mat.

2. Transition into a kneeling position on the bolster, with your feet pointing toward the back of the mat.

3. Slowly lower your body, embracing the bolster, and rest one ear on the side.

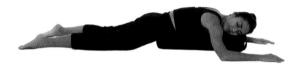

Remain in this pose for up to 15 minutes, remembering to switch to the other ear halfway through.

*This variation of **Shavasana** in the prone position offers a gentle massage-like effect on the abdominal organs, promoting relaxation and alleviating discomfort, which is particularly beneficial for menstrual cramps or digestive issues. As you surrender into the pose, both the upper and lower back receive a subtle stretch, easing tension.*

7
CENTERING

Strength & Core

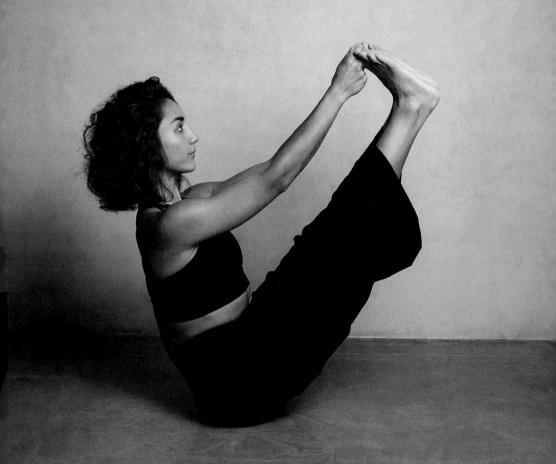

Leg Lifts

1.   Begin in an upright seated position, placing a block flat beneath your buttocks.

2.   Lift your legs one at a time to form a right angle with your upper body, ensuring your knees hover directly above your hips. You may grip the long sides of your mat or firmly press your hands into the floor for support, allowing your shoulders to relax.

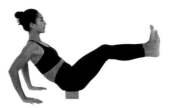

3.   Inhale and lower your right heel toward the mat. Exhale as you lift the leg back to the center.

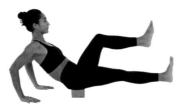

4.   Repeat the sequence on the opposite side.

Complete this sequence on both sides 3–5 times. Afterward, draw your knees toward your chest and take deep breaths into the abdomen.

This exercise is effective for strengthening the abdominal muscles and enhancing hip mobility.

Straight Leg Lifts

1. Lie on your back. Hold a block between your palms and extend your arms overhead.

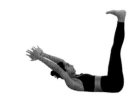

2. Lift your extended legs over your hips, one at a time, ensuring your feet remain flexed.

3. As you exhale, lower your left leg toward the mat, holding the pose for two to three breaths while pressing your hands firmly into the block.

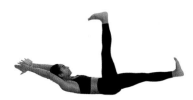

4. Inhale as you lift the leg back to the center, then repeat the sequence on the opposite side.

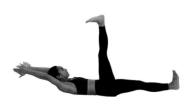

Complete this sequence on both sides three to five times. Afterward, draw your knees toward your chest and take deep breaths into the abdomen.

This challenging exercise targets the core muscles and serves as excellent preparation for handstands. It effectively engages the core and strengthens the entire supporting musculature. However, avoiding this exercise is advisable if you experience pain or discomfort in the lower back.

Side Leg Lifts

1.   Lie on your back and place a block between the thighs.

2.   Lift your legs at a right angle to your upper body.

3.   Position your arms at a right angle, ensuring that your shoulder blades and the back of your hands are grounded.

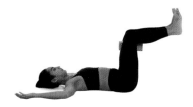

4.   Exhale, lower your legs to the right side while keeping your shoulder blades on the ground.

5.   Inhale, lift your legs back over the hips.

6.   Repeat the sequence on the other side.

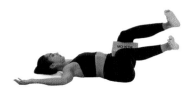

Complete this sequence three to five times on each side. Keep your shoulders as relaxed as possible and lower your legs only as far as you can while maintaining the position of your shoulder blades on the ground.

This exercise is effective for strengthening side trunk muscles.

Standing Balance Exercise

1.   Stand upright, and hold a block in your left hand.

2.   Lift your right leg to a right angle and press the block to the inside of the thigh. Ensure that your foot is flexed and your toes are active.

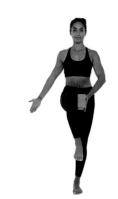

3.   Slowly extend your right arm to the side and return it to the starting position.

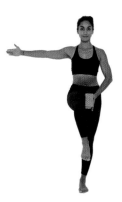

Repeat this sequence five to ten times, maintaining balance while pressing the thigh into the block. Then, repeat the sequence on the other side.

This exercise serves as excellent preparation for all balance exercises. It activates the core and enhances awareness of the deep supporting muscles.

Kakasana—Crow Pose

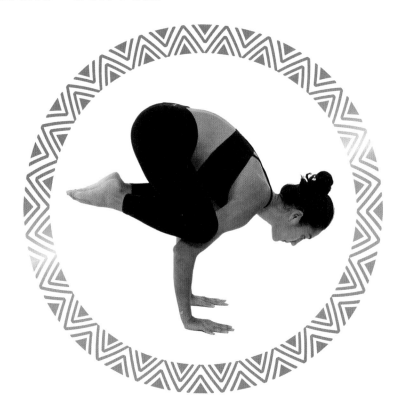

The *Crow Pose* is one of yoga's most well-known arm balance exercises. It requires a lot of courage and overcoming fear, along with strength, flexibility, and balance. The wrists, shoulders, arms, hips, and abdomen muscles are strengthened, especially the core muscles, which need to work intensely to stabilize the body in this pose.

Kakasana is an excellent introduction to other arm balance exercises. Before sufficient holding strength and balance are developed, hip flexibility can be used here by keeping the knees resting on the upper arms.

Kakasana with two blocks

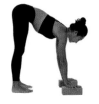

1. Start by placing two flat blocks on either side of the mat.

2. Move into *Uttanasana*, the standing Forward Bend (p. 42).

3. Shift your weight onto the balls of your feet and rest your hands on the blocks.

4. Bend your arms and position your knees on the upper arms.

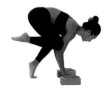

5. Focus the gaze diagonally toward the ground. You may place a blanket in front of you for added support.

6. Press your hands firmly into the blocks and shift your weight into your arms. Lift your right heel toward your buttocks.

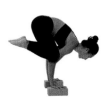

7. Lower the foot back down and repeat the sequence on the other side.

8. Aim to lift both feet off the ground and draw the heels toward your buttocks.

Hold this pose for a few calm breaths while maintaining balance.

This variation is an excellent preparatory exercise to develop balance for the full arm balance pose.

Bakasana—Crane Pose

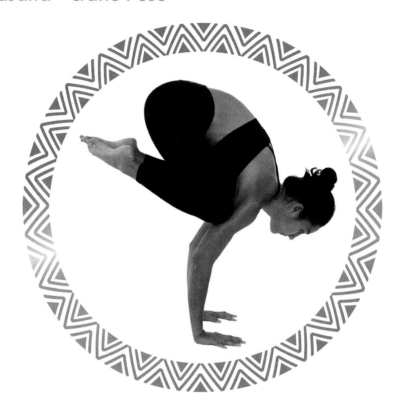

Barkasana or Crane Pose is, in a way, the advanced version of Crow Pose. Unlike *Kakasana*, the arms are fully extended, requiring much more strength. The weight is shifted into the hands, demanding joint stability and strength in the core and upper back.

Ensure wrists are well warmed up before attempting. Avoid the pose if there are wrist issues.

Bakasana with two blocks

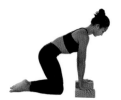

1. Get into Tabletop position with your hands placed firmly on two flat blocks.

2. Press your hands firmly into the blocks, engaging your upper arms and shoulders.

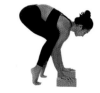

3. Roll your pubic bone toward your navel to engage your core.

4. Draw the belly in and lift the ribcage, coming onto your tiptoes, and round the upper back. Bring your thighs close to your body, ensuring your knees touch the upper arms.

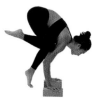

5. Shift more weight into your hands and lift the right heel toward your buttocks.

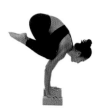

6. Holding the weight with your arms, lift the left foot off the mat, pulling the heels closer to your buttocks. Maintain straight arms throughout.

Hold this pose for several deep breaths, then slowly lower the legs toward the floor while relaxing the shoulders.

*Raising the blocks makes lifting the legs easier until enough core strength is developed. In **Crane Pose**, connecting the thighs to the upper body is essential to ensure a compact core. The blocks act as an extension of the arms, creating additional space to draw the legs closer.*

Steps 1 to 4 target the core before sufficient strength is built in the arms and upper back, making this variation an ideal preparation for the full pose.

Bakasana with a block

1. Place a flat block at the end of the mat.

2. Get into a deep squat with your back turned to the block.

3. Place your toes on the block.

4. Rise higher on the balls of your feet and slightly bend your arms.

5. Place the knees on the upper arms.

6. Press your hands firmly into the mat and shift the weight forward.

7. Keep your gaze diagonally ahead, focused on one point on the floor. You can place a blanket in front of you.

8. Shift more weight into the hands and lift one foot at a time.

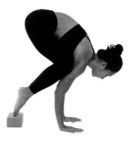

Repeat the sequence several times on both sides.

*The elevation of the feet reduces the distance between the thighs and upper arms. In addition to arm and core strength, **Bakasana** requires significant hip flexor strength to keep the legs as close to the upper body as possible.*

8

EXPERT
Profiles

Cornelius Feist

Yoga teacher (500+ hours) as well as movement teacher at his school Movement Practice in Hamburg. Therapeutic work as an osteopath (1350+ hours) and physiotherapist in his clinic in Hamburg-Altona.

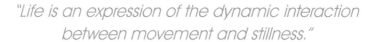

"Life is an expression of the dynamic interaction between movement and stillness."

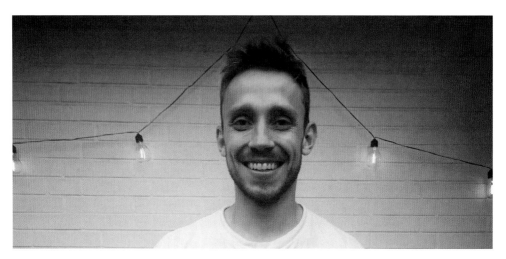

Cornelius is passionate about teaching health and movement in his seminars, teacher training courses, and regular classes. He emphasizes the connection between functional anatomy and physiology and practical empirical sciences such as yoga and movement. Since 2023, he has been training future movement teachers through a one-year Movement Teacher Training course that includes 300 hours of movement practice and theory. The Movement Practice (300 hours MTT) is the first face-to-face didactic movement teacher training in Europe.

Learn more about Cornelius's work:

www.osteopath-hamburg.com (Clinic-Website)
www.movementpractice.de (Movement Practice@)
@cornelius_motus (Instagram)
Seminar, cooperation, and workshop inquiries to:
info@cornelius-feist.com

Maike Lüders

Physiotherapist in Manual and Sports Physiotherapy.

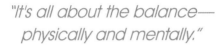

*"It's all about the balance—
physically and mentally."*

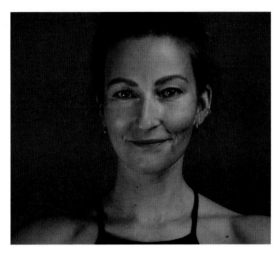

Since 2011, Maike has been a physiotherapist specializing in manual and sports physiotherapy. She focuses on guiding athletes, corporations, and individuals toward better health. Leveraging her extensive rehabilitation and pain management expertise, she crafts personalized plans to help clients seamlessly incorporate health-oriented activities such as yoga into their routines. "The success of a treatment depends significantly on the awareness of how closely the body and mind are connected. Targeted exercises can help develop an understanding of the interaction between physical and mental health."

Learn more about Maike's work:

www.Healthcare-ML.de
Request an appointment:
luedersmaike@gmail.com

Acknowledgments

Completing the first book project—what an accomplishment!

I can still vividly recall the moment when I held Martina Mittag's inspiring *Hatha Yoga* book in my hands, having been a part of the project as a model for Meyer & Meyer. Four years later, while journeying home after a yoga event in Austria, thoughts swirled in my mind about what my inaugural book would be about.

Without hesitation, I reached out to Martina, and her prompt suggestion for a topic immediately resonated with me. In the following weeks and months, a vision for a comprehensive work, unlike anything seen before, began to take shape. Today, as I hold my book in my hands, I am grateful to Martina for her inspiration, collaboration, and support even before this book baby was born.

A heartfelt thank you is also owed to Meyer & Meyer, whose openness and trust in my authorship fueled this collaboration from the start. Special recognition goes to project managers Alexa Deutz and René Kirchhoff, as well as to Robert Meyer.

From the outset, it was clear that the book's essence would be brought to life primarily through its imagery. The quality of the photos and the visual storytelling capturing the essence of yoga were paramount, and photographer Lena Scherer brought my vision to life with precision. I am deeply grateful for our creative and structured collaboration, which resulted in such stunning imagery.

Of course, none of this would have been possible without the foundational groundwork. My heartfelt appreciation goes to my friend, colleague, and physiotherapist Maike Lüders, whose energetic support and expertise were invaluable during the conceptualization phase, instilling confidence in me to convey the essence of safe and well-rounded yoga practice to readers.

I also thank my yoga teacher, colleague, and children's book author, Hanna Gorzinski, who graciously served as my test yogi for pose alignment and prop usage. Our laughter-filled work against the backdrop of Córdoba's magnificent mountains and our Free Spirits Yoga Retreat in Andalusia will always be cherished memories.

In the same vein, I express my appreciation to my osteopath, yoga teacher colleague, and universal specialist Cornelius Feist, whose extensive knowledge of the human body served as a wellspring of inspiration. I trust that your (rightfully!) discerning eye is satisfied with the outcome. Thank you for sharing your remarkable expertise.

Thanks are also due to the contributors of this book: VIO YOGA. A yoga equipment manufacturer and cooperation partner, they provided all yoga straps, blocks, and bolsters featured throughout the book.

A heartfelt thank you to Hey Honey for their generous provision of black yoga leggings and sports bras, which afforded me great comfort during the shoots.

And, of course, many thanks to OH Rodzinski OM ethical sportswear, who outfitted me with my favorite black top and a relaxed ensemble for the Yin and Restorative images.

Special gratitude goes out to dear Simone Leuschner for the photos captured after the conceptualization of the book content and for the author's portrait showcased on the last pages of this book. Your work in Focus on Yoga is truly remarkable!

Sara Lyn Chana

The author

"Yoga is the connection
with and to ourselves."

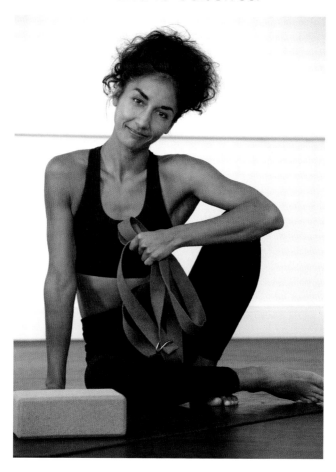

Sara Lyn Chana is a certified yoga instructor, Pilates trainer, and state-certified specialist journalist. Her fascination with the human body and graceful movement patterns started twenty-five years ago at the ballet barre. Despite opting for a conventional academic route after high school instead of pursuing formal dance training, Sara Lyn concurrently trained to become a Pilates teacher. After completing her sociology degree, she embarked on a nine-month journey across Asia and her second home—Thailand. Throughout her travels, her faithful companion was nothing more than a backpack—and a yoga mat!

Sara Lyn began her yoga journey by mastering poses from a book, diligently practicing every morning. Once she felt confident in her practice, she set her sights on India. During her journalistic studies, she ventured to distant Goa for a 200-hour teacher training, immersing herself in various yoga styles like Hatha, Ashtanga, and Vinyasa.

Back in Germany, she seized every opportunity to teach. Seven days a week, she embarked on a pilgrimage through Hamburg's studios to further her education. Only two years later, her spiritual quest led her back to the roots of yoga. In 2017 she completed an intense 300-hour Hatha and Ashtanga training in Rishikesh, nestled in the Himalayas. After the six-week intensive training in the mountains of North India, she had the opportunity to expand her passion for martial arts and traditional Muay Thai in Thailand further. This gave her a better understanding of working with dancers and martial artists.

Sara Lyn's goal is to encourage her students based on their individual needs and strengths. In her Online Coaching Programs, she designs personal programs for her clients in order to support them on their journey to more strength, flexibility, and self-consciousness—not only physically, but also mentally. For a deeper movement experience and understanding of the mental background of her teachings, she runs several retreats and teacher trainings per year to connect with her students in person and in special places, mostly Europe and Asia.

You can find all her online programs, coaching, and training on her official website: www.saralynyoga.com

And on social media:

 @saralyn.yoga

 Sara Lyn

 www.saralyn.de

References

Iyengar, B. K. S. (1966). *Licht auf Yoga* (Light on Yoga). *Das grundlegende Lehrbuch des Hatha-Yoga.* München: O. W. Barth Verlag.

Iyengar, B.K.S. (2014). *Yoga – der Weg zu Gesundheit und Harmonie.* München: Dorling Kindersley.

Mittag, M. (2018). *Hatha Yoga – das komplette Buch.* Aachen: Meyer & Meyer.

Shifroni, E. (2015). *Props for Yoga – Volume 1: Standing Poses.* Createspace Independent Publishing Platform.

Shifroni, E. (2016). *Props for Yoga – Volume 2*: Sitting Asanas and Forward Extensions. Createspace Independent Publishing Platform.

Skuban, R. (2011). *Patanjalis Yogasutra – Der Königsweg zu einem weisen Leben* (7. Auflage). München: Arkana Verlag.

Neuber, L. (2019). *Restorative Yoga.* München: Südwest Verlag.

Credits

Cover design: Annika Naas, Anja Elsen

Interior design: Isabella Frangenberg

Layout: Anja Elsen

Cover and interior photos: Lena Scherer Fotografie, www.lenascherer.de

Chapter 2 figures: p. 18-19 © AdobeStock

Managing editor: Elizabeth Evans

Translator: Mirjam Schmidt

Copy editor: Sarah Tomblin, www.sarahtomblinediting.com